The Morehouse Mystique

THE MOREHOUSE
MYSTIQUE

Becoming a Doctor at the Nation's Newest
African American Medical School

MARYBETH GASMAN

with LOUIS W. SULLIVAN

Foreword by Barbara Bush

The Johns Hopkins University Press

Baltimore

© 2012 The Johns Hopkins University Press
All rights reserved. Published 2012
Printed in the United States of America on acid-free paper
2 4 6 8 9 7 5 3 1

The Johns Hopkins University Press
2715 North Charles Street
Baltimore, Maryland 21218-4363
www.press.jhu.edu

Library of Congress Cataloging-in-Publication Data

Gasman, Marybeth.
The Morehouse mystique : becoming a doctor at the nation's newest African American
medical school / Marybeth Gasman ; with Louis W. Sullivan ; foreword by Barbara Bush.
p. cm.
Includes bibliographical references and index.
ISBN-13: 978-1-4214-0443-1 (hdbk. : alk. paper)
ISBN-10: 1-4214-0443-5 (hdbk. : alk. paper)
ISBN-13: 978-1-4214-0604-6 (electronic)
ISBN-10: 1-4214-0604-7 (electronic)
1. Morehouse School of Medicine.   2. African American medical colleges—
Georgia.   3. Medical colleges—Georgia.   I. Sullivan, Louis Wade, 1933–   II. Title.
R747.M87G37 2012
610.71'1758—dc23   2011026542

A catalog record for this book is available from the British Library.

*Special discounts are available for bulk purchases of this book. For more information, please
contact Special Sales at 410-516-6936 or specialsales@press.jhu.edu.*

The Johns Hopkins University Press uses environmentally friendly book materials,
including recycled text paper that is composed of at least 30 percent post-consumer
waste, whenever possible.

We call that something the "Morehouse Mystique." The phrase is not easily defined or understood, but it's also not just a clever slogan. The Mystique is joining a brotherhood like none other. And after being ignored, stereotyped, or marginalized, it's about finally finding that "home" that, deep inside, you always knew existed, where you are the heart, soul, and hope of the community. And where you are not alone.

Morehouse College

The tragedy of life doesn't lie in not reaching your goal. The tragedy lies in having no goals to reach.

Benjamin E. Mays
President of Morehouse College
1940–1967

Future historians will likely judge that the most important contribution of Morehouse College since its founding was the launching of the nation's third predominantly Black medical school.

Hugh M. Gloster
President of Morehouse College
1967–1987

CONTENTS

Morehouse School of Medicine has made a profound difference in the lives of countless people. It fills a unique niche in medical education by training doctors who care about low-income and minority patients. I am so proud of the school's remarkable accomplishments and am grateful to have been a part of it during the beginning.

I became involved with Morehouse School of Medicine when my husband was vice president of the United States. In November 1982, George led a delegation on a trip to Sub-Saharan Africa, and the group included the talented Dr. Louis Sullivan. I enjoyed getting to know Lou on this trip and learning about Morehouse. The school was started to train doctors—men and women—to return to underserved urban and rural areas that had little or no medical care. Sullivan's dedication to training minority doctors, who would then go out into the world to care for those most in need, was truly inspirational. Shortly after we returned from Africa, he invited me to join Morehouse School of Medicine's Board of Directors. I accepted and spent six very happy years with some of the finest men and women.

Morehouse is now a top producer of African American health professionals, and their alumni are wonderfully impressive. For example, just recently, Morehouse alumna Regina Benjamin was awarded the MacArthur "Genius" Award and was chosen to be the nineteenth Surgeon General of the United States Public Health Service.

It is not easy to start and support a medical school. Louis Sullivan did it—and he did it very well. This book chronicles the interesting history of Morehouse, highlighting the exciting and challenging time during its development. In these pages, readers will learn how Louis Sullivan, with the help of Morehouse students, faculty, administrators, alumni, and trustees, brought the school from a high-risk idea to a successful reality. Readers will also come to understand the important role Morehouse School of Medicine plays in the history of major African American accomplishments.

Barbara Bush

In fall 2007 I received a call from Marc Nivet, chief financial officer at the Josiah Macy Jr. Foundation. He had just read my book *Envisioning Black Colleges* and, thankfully, he enjoyed it. Nivet asked whether I would be interested in writing a history of Morehouse School of Medicine, which the foundation was funding. He put me in touch with Louis W. Sullivan, the school's president emeritus, who was spearheading the project, and soon I began the research that led to this book. Working with Lou has been a joy. He has a terrific sense of humor and a memory for wonderful stories. Perhaps what I appreciated most is that Lou wanted the medical school's entire story told—the strengths and the challenges. For me, a serious history was essential to depicting this important institution.

Writing the history of an institution is a large endeavor, drawn from the memories and perspectives of many individuals. For this project, I relied on the help of several people. First, Kijua Sanders McMurtry served as my research assistant and combed through stacks of papers to find evidence that I could use to build the story of Morehouse School of Medicine. Kijua is a superb historian, doing work on African American philanthropy and social service organizations. Her perspective and keen eye were invaluable. I also had the pleasure of working with several other research assistants, including Julie Vultaggio, who researched the alumni profiles in the book's appendix; Darryl L. Peterkin, who investigated the medical school's relationship with Grady Hospital; Valerie Lundy Wagner, who helped me gather statistics on medical education for African Americans; Christopher Tudico, who pulled materials on the medical school's relationship with the Josiah Macy Jr. Foundation; Thai-Huy Nguyen, who secured the interview permissions and compiled the index; and Tafaya Ransom and Esther Ra, who read early drafts of the manuscript. I am incredibly lucky to have talented research assistants who are interested in African American higher education and, specifically, Black colleges and universities. Each of them is pursuing his or her own research as well, and I look forward to seeing how they change the field of higher education. In addition to these research assistants, I was assisted by Jonathan Wallace on the manuscript. He is a superb editor.

I am also grateful to those affiliated with Morehouse School of Medicine who helped me gather information for this book. Gayle McDaniels, the administrative assistant to Louis W. Sullivan, was invaluable and joyful. Others who helped pull archival materials, gather photographs, and put me in connection with alumni and key actors in the medical school story included Gayle Converse, Cynthia Henderson, Mary Kay Murphy, Yolanda Sapp, and Carrie Dumas.

Ashleigh McKown and Jacqueline Wehmueller, our editors at the Johns Hopkins University Press, believed in this project and shepherded it throughout our writing and editing process. I am thankful to them for thoughtfully pushing us to do our best work.

I thank my friends and family for their support while I was writing this book. My colleagues at the University of Pennsylvania contribute to a wonderful environment in which to do research. Two close friends, in particular, listened to much of my thinking about this project over the past couple of years. I am grateful to Noah D. Drezner and Nelson Bowman III for helping me think through aspects of this book and for their sense of humor. Lastly, my inspiration for any scholarly project and for all that I do in life is drawn from my sweet, sweet daughter Chloe Sarah Epstein.

Marybeth Gasman

Every day of my life I have learned something new, or gained a new and valuable insight. Writing the history of Morehouse School of Medicine with Marybeth Gasman has been, for me, one of those learning experiences. Her discipline as a historian, combined with her enthusiasm and scholarship, has made this a joyous undertaking.

It is not possible for me to acknowledge all of those to whom I am indebted. However, I do wish to note those who have contributed most significantly to my efforts to develop Morehouse School of Medicine—truly a team effort. First are my parents, Walter Sullivan Sr. and Lubirda Priester Sullivan. They instilled in me an unending thirst for knowledge and challenged me to use that knowledge to help make a better world—for me and for others. Then there was Dr. Joseph Griffin of Bainbridge, Georgia, the only Black physician in the southwest corner of rural Georgia where I grew up—he was my first physician role model. My teachers at Booker T. Washington High School in Atlanta worked very hard to see that I and my classmates mastered our academic work and participated in events to enrich our community, such as the marching band, the chorus, and athletic events.

My high school heroes include my ninth-grade teacher, Ms. Laura Woods; my eighth-grade geometry teacher, Mr. Martin; my tenth-grade chemistry teacher, Mr. X. L. Neal; my eleventh-grade English teacher, Mr. A. R. Phillips; and many others. At Morehouse College, I was inspired by the eloquence of President Benjamin E. Mays and his strong value system, and by James Birnie, professor of biology. In fact, I was constantly amazed and challenged by my professors in chemistry, mathematics, the social sciences, and the humanities, who broadened my vision of the world and its infinite possibilities. My enrollment at Boston University School of Medicine opened a new chapter for me, living for the first time in a non-segregated environment. My medical school professors and my classmates were supportive, challenging, and inspiring, which stimulated me to achieve even more. As a student, and later as an intern and a research fellow, I was fortunate to interact with some of the intellectual giants in medicine: Chester Keefer, Franz Ingelfinger, Arnold Relman, E. Hugh Luckey, David Rogers, William Castle, Maxwell Finland, Victor Herbert, and others.

All of these interactions, and what I learned from these mentors, helped prepare me for the challenge and the opportunity of serving as the founding dean of Morehouse School of Medicine—the only predominantly Black four-year medical school founded in the United States in the twentieth century. Helping me bring this concept to fruition was a host of individuals and organizations, as well as an improving racial and social climate in our country, led by the civil rights movement.

Atlanta physician Dr. Louis Brown was a visionary who persisted and succeeded in his efforts to convince people that a new medical school was needed and could be developed at the Atlanta University Center. Hugh M. Gloster, president of Morehouse College, responded to the challenge and founded Morehouse School of Medicine—a unique challenge for an undergraduate college. Supporting President Gloster's efforts were Calvin A. Brown, MD, vice-chairman of the Board of Trustees of Morehouse College, and three college faculty members—Joseph V. Gayles, Thomas R. Norris, and Alice G. Greene. These four were advised by William Bennett, a program director in the Bureau of Health Manpower of the U.S. Public Health Service. Helping to guide this medical education initiative was a Board of Overseers, formed in April 1976 and led by Edgar Smith (chairman), Monroe Trout (vice-chairman), and Sarah Austin (secretary). Dean Arthur Richardson of Emory University School of Medicine gave his active support to the effort, along with Garland Herndon (vice president for health affairs), Bernard Hall-man (associate dean), Jonas Schulman, Charles Hatcher, and Asa Yancy (medical director of Grady Hospital), all at Emory School of Medicine. Rhodes Haverty, MD, president of the Georgia State Medical Association, provided guidance and secured the endorsement of the Medical Association of Georgia (a state affiliate of the American Medical Association), complementing the support of the Georgia State Medical Association (a state affiliate of the National Medical Association).

Working closely with me to help in the transition of my professional career from teaching and research to administration and policy was Stanley Olson, former dean of Baylor College of Medicine. At first, Stan was a planning consultant who wrote "The Path Ahead," the strategic plan for Morehouse School of Medicine's transition from a two-year to a four-year medical school. In 1983, when we separated the positions of president and dean, Stan became dean of Morehouse School of Medicine, serving until 1985.

In the development of Morehouse School of Medicine, its students and faculty members have played—and continue to play—a central role. Although Morehouse School of Medicine became independent from Morehouse College on July 1, 1981, the alumni of Morehouse College, great supporters from the beginning, continue to be active proponents of the institution. Finally, I owe an infinite measure of love and gratitude to my wife, Ginger, for her enduring, enthusiastic support of all my endeavors, and for being the center of gravity for our family, including our children, Paul, Shanta, and Halsted.

The history of Morehouse School of Medicine shows that significant things can be accomplished if they are supported by an ever-growing group of individuals, working together in common purpose, bringing with them their different talents and perspectives, and blending them into a symphony that never before existed.

Louis W. Sullivan, MD

The Morehouse Mystique

Introduction

For more than a century, the United States has vigorously debated how to provide medical care to the greatest number of people. Politicians, interest groups, and ordinary citizens—in an effort to guarantee access to health care for the millions of Americans who are without it—have argued over whether to adopt a European-style system of socialized medicine or to tinker with the existing system of private insurance. Lost in the din is the fact that minority citizens—African Americans, in particular—are among those least well cared for in the United States. Their rates of infant mortality are higher, their life expectancy is shorter, and they suffer from higher rates of many ailments, such as heart disease, cancer, stroke, and diabetes.[1] According to a 2004 Institute of Medicine report, *Unequal Treatment: Confronting Racial and Ethnic Disparities in Health Care*, "racial and ethnic health care disparities [exist] even when insurance status, age, income and illness severity [are] taken into account."[2] Contributing to this problem is African Americans' lack of access to primary care and prenatal care: they often live in impoverished communities with a shortage of doctors.

Why the shortage? One explanation is that, in the past, fewer African Americans had the opportunity to become doctors, and of those who did, only a small percentage returned to their communities to care for those most in need. The *Unequal Treatment* report also suggests that although the majority of "health professionals dedicate themselves to providing the highest quality of care possible to every patient, they also might harbor unconscious biases and stereotypes that affect their decision-making and attitudes toward minority patients."[3] Many mainstream medical schools have neglected to provide their graduates with cultural competence—a sensitivity to racial and ethnic differences—in terms of health care. Likewise, they have failed to instill in their graduates a dedication to social responsibility and community outreach.[4]

This book tells the story of one institution, Morehouse School of Medicine, that was founded, in part, to correct Blacks' lack of access to medical education and medical care, and that places an emphasis on cultural competence and providing health care to people who are underserved. According to a recent study in the *Annals of Internal Medicine*, Morehouse ranks first among U.S. medical schools in terms of its social mission to the community, followed by two other historically Black medical schools. On the other hand, institutions with a heavy research emphasis, including the most prestigious medical schools in the nation, scored near the very bottom on social mission.[5]

The American Medical Association (AMA) has acknowledged African Americans' continued and historic lack of access to and, in fact, systemic exclusion from medical education and medical careers. In July 2008, following an AMA-appointed expert panel's report on the history of racial division in American medicine,[6] AMA president Ronald M. Davis, a young, forward-thinking physician, formally apologized on behalf of the organization. In particular, Davis apologized for the AMA's history of excluding African American physicians from its membership rolls, of identifying Black doctors as "colored" in its national directory of physicians, of neglecting to speak out against federal funding of segregated hospitals, and of failing to support civil rights activities and legislation.[7] Denial of membership in the AMA had many ramifications. For example, African American doctors had to forgo income and prestige because they could rarely get hospital privileges without AMA membership. Most Blacks went into private practice, with very low-income patients, because they could not secure hospital residencies. Davis pledged that the AMA would "do everything in [its] power to right the wrongs that were done by [the] organization to African American physicians and their families and their patients."[8] In making his statement, Davis recognized that the AMA apology was merely a "modest first step toward healing and reconciliation" around issues of race and medicine.[9]

To rectify its past exclusionary practices, the AMA and its membership have developed several initiatives to increase the number of African American doctors. For example, the AMA's Minority Affairs Consortium developed a program called Doctors Back to School, which has sent doctors into schools to talk with more than 13,000 students from underrepresented groups about careers in medicine. In addition, the AMA awards over $100,000 to minority medical students every year—a paltry sum, but at least a start.[10]

According to Larry Cuban, the author of *How Scholars Trumped Teachers*, medical education traditionally has focused on technical proficiency, public service, scientific discovery, and staying up to date about new knowledge and procedures.[11] The AMA has agreed to add another goal to that focus: raising physicians' awareness of disparities and of the importance of understanding culturally competent health care.[12] It aims to close gaps in access to proper medical care by working with state medical societies, medical schools, students, and those trying to change policy.[13] This kind of approach is essential, given the history of exclusion of African Americans at all levels of medicine and medical education.

A Medical School Begins

Morehouse School of Medicine was born during a period of great expansion in medical education in the United States. One reason for this growth was the recognition of a national shortage of physicians during the 1950s.[14] From 1956 to 1981, owing to federal legislation and state financial support, forty-seven new medical schools were established, or one in every three U.S. medical schools today.[15]

Morehouse School of Medicine is the only predominantly Black four-year medical school founded in the United States in the twentieth century, and it is one of only four predominantly Black medical schools.[16] Meharry Medical College and Howard University are both four-year institutions founded in the nineteenth century; Charles R. Drew School of Medicine, a two-year institution, was founded in 1966 as an affiliate of the University of California, Los Angeles (UCLA). The idea of Morehouse School of Medicine began in 1969 with the advocacy of Louis Brown, a Black doctor in Atlanta. Brown served on a committee appointed by the Georgia Comprehensive Health Planning Council to evaluate the state's physician manpower. The committee documented a shortage of Black physicians. With support from the Georgia State Medical Association (a state affiliate of the historically Black National Medical Association) and from the Medical Association of Georgia (a state affiliate of the formerly White American Medical Association), Brown proposed the idea of starting a medical school to Atlanta University, which served as the graduate school for the Atlanta University Center, a consortium of six historically Black higher education institutions. President Thomas Jarrett and the Board of Trustees of Atlanta University, however, thought the idea was too risky. Instead, the forward-thinking president of Morehouse College, Hugh Gloster, expressed interest, and that interest blossomed over the next decade.

On July 1, 1975, with the appointment of Louis W. Sullivan, MD, as dean and director of the Medical Education Program, Morehouse School of Medicine was founded. Its mission was the "education and training of more physicians from minority and socioeconomically disadvantaged groups for work as primary care physicians for our medically underserved citizens in rural areas and inner cities."[17] This mission drew a groundswell of support, as well as some controversy, from the Atlanta and Georgia communities.[18]

Atlanta and the South as a Backdrop

The South was in the midst of the turbulent civil rights era. African Americans protesting in Birmingham, Alabama, in 1963 were viciously suppressed. As a result, the people of United States and the world became more aware of the brutality against Blacks in the South.[19] Widespread knowledge of this event helped build sympathy for civil rights and assisted then president Lyndon Johnson in passing a series of important pieces of legislation, including the 1964 Civil Rights Act. The Civil Rights Act gave Congress broad powers to prevent discrimination in public accommodations and schools. This legislation had an effect in Georgia, where the Medical College of Georgia still excluded Black students in 1964.

In 1965 the world watched as hundreds of Black and White citizens attempted to march from Selma, Alabama, to Montgomery, Alabama, to support the tenets of the Civil Rights Act, including voting rights for Blacks. They were savagely attacked by angry White mobs.[20] Soon after the bloody Sunday event, in which Alabama state troopers attacked peaceful protestors, Congress enacted the Voting Rights Act of 1965. This legislation finally eliminated barriers that had prevented Blacks from voting in the South and all but ensured that some cities would be governed by a Black majority. Along with congressional acts in favor of peaceful protest, the courts began to support equality for African Americans in significant ways, ruling that civil rights protesters had the lawful right to voice their dissatisfaction.[21]

These national events had direct repercussions in Georgia and in the city of Atlanta. As a result of the Voting Rights Act, African American Julian Bond was elected to be a legislator in the state house of representatives in 1965, but the Georgia General Assembly refused to seat him, in part because he supported Vietnam-era conscientious objectors.[22] Bond was eventually reelected in 1966 and, by an order of the United States Supreme Court, allowed to join his fellow legislators later that year. Though some Georgia Whites supported Bond, race relations remained tense.

The city of Atlanta played a complex role in the success of Morehouse School of Medicine. As countless historians have demonstrated, the "city too busy to hate" experienced race riots, segregation, and discrimination. In

1965, a future governor of Georgia, Lester Maddox (who would serve from 1967 to 1971), was ordered to desegregate his Pickrick Restaurant or close it; for several years, the restaurant had been the scene of protests and assaults on Blacks. Maddox chose to close it—an indication of the reaction of some White segregationists in Atlanta against the concept of equality of the races.[23] The citizens of Georgia elected segregationist Maddox in one of the tightest gubernatorial races in the state's history. It took 47 percent of the state's residents, the state legislature, and a ruling from the U.S. Supreme Court to move Maddox into office—setting the state back in terms of its race relations once again.[24] Still, there were people in Atlanta who saw that Blacks and Whites could work together to build the city and make it a center of finance and commerce in the South and across the nation.

Following the passage of landmark civil rights legislation, the country's support for civil rights wavered. Across the nation, racial unrest was bubbling up in cities such as Tampa, Florida, Buffalo, New York, Newark, New Jersey, Detroit, Michigan, and Washington, D.C.[25] Hundreds of protesters, Black and White, were injured or killed, and buildings and businesses were burned. Atlanta became the scene of racial violence as well, with riots erupting in the Summerhill neighborhood on September 6, 1966.

A hopeful event took place on the federal level when, in 1967, President Johnson nominated Thurgood Marshall, U.S. solicitor general and former general counsel for the National Association for the Advancement of Colored People (NAACP) Legal Defense Fund, to be the first African American Supreme Court associate justice. Still, there was discomfort with equality for Blacks throughout the land.[26] In April 1968, Martin Luther King Jr., a son of Atlanta, was shot and killed the day after delivering his "I've been to the mountaintop" speech in Memphis, Tennessee. The civil rights leader's death prompted more riots in major American cities.[27] In Atlanta, Governor Maddox refused to close state government offices in tribute to King, nor did he attend King's funeral. Maddox viewed the civil rights leader as an "enemy of the country" and treated King's mourners and supporters as enemies as well. The segregationist governor even stationed more than 50 state police officers dressed in riot gear outside the state capitol to protect state property during the funeral.[28]

But as former president Jimmy Carter would later say, Atlanta was "probably the most enlightened part of Georgia."[29] Carter thought that the city's more cosmopolitan outlook was in part due to the influence of the *Atlanta Journal-Constitution* newspaper, which had a very progressive editorial staff.

Carter became governor of Georgia after Maddox had served one term. "When I ran for governor," Carter said, "I could detect the presence of a racial divide quite deeply throughout the state. When I was elected governor in 1971, I made an inaugural address and said, quite frankly, that the time for racial discrimination is over, and never again will a Black child be deprived of an equal right to health care and education and other social advantages of life. That was kind of a startling thing to say in January of 1971." Just a few weeks later, Carter was on the front cover of *Time* magazine because of his inaugural address remarks.

Change was slow in Georgia overall. Carter recalled that when he decided to hang a portrait of Martin Luther King Jr. in the state capitol, "the Ku Klux Klan marched around the capital all during the ceremony with their white robes, but I went ahead, of course, and did it." It was in such a climate of racial tension that the idea for Morehouse School of Medicine was born.

This book tells the story of the creation and development of Morehouse School of Medicine, situating it within the larger expansion of medical education for Blacks and of race relations in Atlanta and the nation. It chronicles a diverse group of African American leaders whose aim was to change the landscape of medical education and the racial and ethnic makeup of physicians and the health professions. The book is organized into eight chapters and includes an appendix focused on the accomplishments of the school's alumni. It is written chronologically, while also focusing on three central themes: strong mission, determined leadership, and interracial cooperation. Morehouse School of Medicine, from its beginnings to the current day, has held fast to its mission of preparing African American doctors and those who are eager to serve in rural and urban areas that have great need. One of the hallmarks of the medical school's history thus far is its strong and ambitious presidential leadership, which has sustained the institution but has also served as a distraction on occasion, taking the focus off the medical school's main goal of educating primary care doctors. The other characteristic of the institution's history is its foundation on interracial cooperation. In a city and state that are known for racial unrest, Morehouse School of Medicine stands as an example of Blacks and Whites coming together to support a common cause.

Chapter 1 provides background on African Americans and medical education in the United States, exploring the development of Black medical schools as well as the experiences of African Americans in historically White medical schools. The chapter also covers the role of philanthropy in the education of

African American doctors, racial discrimination, and legal barriers to equitable higher education.

Chapter 2 discusses the birth of Morehouse School of Medicine, highlighting the situation for Black doctors and Black citizens in Georgia and across the nation. Notably, it explores the arguments for and against the medical school from the perspective of both the Black and the White communities in Georgia. The chapter also discusses the role that the federal government played in developing Morehouse School of Medicine, as well as the school's unique collaboration with Emory University and other medical schools.

Chapter 3 focuses on initial fundraising efforts, as well as on how the campus first developed under Sullivan's leadership. Chapter 4 chronicles the school's coming into its own—as it grew from a two-year to a four-year institution and became fully accredited. These accomplishments were made possible through strategic state and federal collaborations and hard work on the part of faculty, staff, leadership, and community members. In many ways, the discussion in these two chapters serves as a model for developing an institution. The Morehouse College administration reached out to multiple and diverse constituencies in order to build the medical school, and there is much to be learned from their strategies.

When Sullivan left to serve as Secretary of the U.S. Department of Health and Human Services in the George H. W. Bush administration, Morehouse School of Medicine's strength was tested. Could it flourish without its founding leader? As demonstrated in chapter 5, it did so under two transitional presidents, James Goodman and Nelson McGhee, who maintained the direction Sullivan had set forth—a direction characterized by interracial cooperation, strong fundraising, and growing enrollment.

Chapter 6 explores the turmoil that ensued when a new leader stepped in with his own strong vision of how to run Morehouse School of Medicine and interact with the Atlanta community. This vision differed distinctly from Sullivan's. James Gavin, although well liked by the faculty, staff, and students, could not get sufficient backing for his agenda at the institution, and the Board of Trustees eventually asked him to leave. Support for the institution, from both the Black and the White communities, wavered during this tumultuous period. The divisions that appeared throughout Gavin's administration exemplify the difficulties faced by founder-driven institutions. Moreover, this chapter, as well as chapter 7, offers a word of caution to new institutional leaders who want to establish themselves on a founder-driven campus. Likewise, these chapters offer commentary on the role of boards of trustees in institutional leadership and governance.

Fortunately, Morehouse School of Medicine's internal cohesion allowed it to withstand the turmoil of President Gavin's administration. As chapter 7 explains, under the leadership of David Satcher and John Maupin, the institution emerged with a sense of strength and determination to move forward in pursuit of its mission. Not only did the medical school renew its national accreditation and increase its viability as a research institution, it also strengthened its fundraising infrastructure.

Chapter 8 examines how students at the medical school interacted with the faculty and administration. Their experiences shed light on the unique Black college environment, showing how faculty both nurture and challenge their students. The book concludes with a chapter that brings together the contributions of Morehouse School of Medicine with the opportunities and obstacles that African Americans face today and in the future. The conclusion examines the strengths and weaknesses of the school, while also exploring the challenges that the medical school will face in the future. And the appendix highlights prominent alumni—including Regina Benjamin, the U.S. Surgeon General under President Barack Obama—with an eye toward the contributions these alumni made to society and to their alma mater.

This book illuminates an important period in the history of medicine and medical education in the United States. From the Morehouse story, we learn how a small yet dedicated group of doctors and educators was able to rally support across racial and political lines to bring greater equity and access to the medical profession. We hear about the difficulties of the enterprise—the battles lost as well as won—and how, over the years, Morehouse leaders were able to overcome those difficulties to build a vibrant and successful institution. It is a story about how race and politics intersected with higher education during the aftermath of the civil rights era—how old practices were sometimes overturned and new allegiances formed. Most importantly, it is a story about leadership, both among the founders of Morehouse and among its alumni, who, following the example of their teachers and mentors, broke new ground in the medical profession—establishing a school dedicated to primary care and with a social mission.[30]

As Morehouse School of Medicine matures, so does the medical profession in the United States. In 2004, for example, under the leadership of Nancy H. Nielsen of the AMA, Sandra Gadson of the National Medical Association (representing African American doctors), and Elena V. Rios of the

National Hispanic Medical Association, the Commission on Health Disparities took root.[31] The commission's work over the past few years has brought
attention to minorities' unequal access to proper health care. The commission has made headway in initiating and influencing federal, state, and local
policy related to health disparities. This body is also working to increase diversity within the health care profession by fostering opportunities for people
of color. With its emphasis on doctors' cultural competence and on working
in urban and rural communities to increase access to health care, Morehouse
School of Medicine is a key player in reaching the commission's goals. Rural
and urban communities with large concentrations of African Americans
continue to have the lowest physician-to-population ratios.[32] Moreover, this
research shows that African American doctors, as well as other doctors who
belong to racial and ethnic minority groups, are more inclined to have patients of color and that these patients have a greater probability of being on
Medicaid or being uninsured. In addition, minority patients are more likely
to consult a doctor of their own race. Thus African American patients will
receive more timely and effective health care if there are more minority doctors. Morehouse School of Medicine is playing a significant role in educating
these doctors.

African Americans and the Medical Profession

The first known African American who graduated from medical school in the United States was David John Peck, who finished his studies at Benjamin Rush Medical School in 1847. According to Wilbur H. Watson, author of *Against the Odds: Blacks in the Profession of Medicine in the United States,* "the next twelve years following Peck's success witnessed the efforts of several other African Americans and institutions of higher education to pave the way for an increasing presence of blacks in medicine."[1] African Americans who pursued a medical education faced racial discrimination and legal barriers in those early years, which helped lead to the creation and growth of Black medical schools. But the attempted standardization of the medical profession nearly led to their demise.

The Antebellum Years

Between 1848 and 1860, only five institutions admitted or granted medical degrees to African American students. John V. de Grassa graduated from Bowdoin College in Maine in 1849, and Western Homeopathic College of Cleveland, Ohio, conferred an MD on Samuel C. Watson in 1857. In 1860, New England Female Medical College (now Boston University School of Medicine) enrolled Rebecca Lee, who became the first Black female MD in the United States when she graduated in 1864. Two other medical schools admitted African American students, but the students' situations were more complicated. Harvard Medical College, for example, enrolled Martin R. Delany, Daniel Laing, and Isaac H. Snowden in 1850, but, as a result of student and faculty protests over "race mixing," the students were dismissed in 1851. Of the three, only Laing was able to enroll at another institution, Dartmouth College; he graduated in 1854.[2] Although few in number, these achievements by African Americans are significant in that they took place during a time of slavery in the South and widespread discrimination in the North. Notably, all the medical programs that conferred degrees on African Americans, with the exception of the Ohio-based Homeopathic College, were in New England.[3]

Before the Civil War, there were no Black medical schools in the United States. According to Watson: "The earliest documented effort in this regard was undertaken in 1862 by the United Presbyterian Church of Nashville, Tennessee. This church-based institution was founded 'for the purpose of befriending the friendless, homeless Negroes who flocked into Nashville.'"[4] It is not clear whether Blacks actually received any medical degrees under this initiative, but Watson noted that the documents left behind give the impression that there were some graduates.

Medical Education after the War

In the years following the Civil War, White and Black missionaries, as well as the federal government's Freedmen's Bureau, established colleges, primarily in the South, for formerly enslaved Black people. Often these institutions were colleges in name only, offering high school curricula, but they aspired to become colleges in full. These early Black colleges provided both a classical liberal arts education and a practical education that focused on learning a skill and preparing to enter the workforce. In addition, Black colleges emphasized religion, as the missionaries worried that the newly freed Blacks would become a menace to society without strict religious instruction.[5] Interestingly, a few of these pioneer institutions included medical education in their curricula, suggesting that their founders sensed a need for Black physicians to serve the Black population.[6]

According to sociologists Christopher Jencks and David Riesman, in their book *The Academic Revolution*, American medical education during the immediate post–Civil War period was "hopelessly unscientific and ineffective," offering a basic curriculum aimed at undergraduates.[7] It was not until 1893, with the establishment of the Johns Hopkins University Medical School—a graduate medical program—that medicine became more research focused and scientific.[8] Within this haphazard system of medical education, one consistent point was the desire to exclude Blacks. Only a few historically White institutions in the North would, on occasion, take Black medical students, but those in the South refused Blacks entry as a rule. Blacks, therefore, had to create their own medical programs.[9] Notably, Howard University in Washington, D.C., established a medical school in 1868; it was the first medical school below the Mason-Dixon Line to enroll Blacks.[10] Howard accepted both

Black and White students in its medical school, as did most Black colleges (unless forbidden by state law). And, unlike White medical schools, Howard's medical school also accepted women.[11] According to Paul Starr's *The Social Transformation of American Medicine: The Rise of a Sovereign Profession and the Making of a Vast Industry*, although some White medical schools originally had liberal policies toward White women, women were excluded as seats in the schools became more scarce. "Administrators justified outright discrimination against qualified women candidates," Starr says, "on the grounds that they would not continue to practice after marriage."[12]

According to Todd L. Savitt, in his seminal history *Race & Medicine in Nineteenth- and Early Twentieth-Century America*, a few of the Black colleges in the South added medical programs, although these programs were short lived. In 1873, for example, Joseph W. Healy established a program at Straight University in New Orleans. Although some scholars have claimed that this medical program was highly successful, it operated for only a few years, "graduated no physicians, employed a teaching faculty of one, and had quite poor instructional facilities."[13] The program was eventually closed in 1877, both because of a fire that destroyed Straight's main campus and a lack of financial resources.

In 1876 George W. Hubbard created a medical department at Central Tennessee College in Nashville. This program, funded by the Freedmen's Aid Society of the Methodist Episcopal Church, would eventually become Meharry Medical College.[14] In 1882 the American Baptist Home Mission Society, under the leadership of Henry M. Tupper, opened Leonard Medical School of Shaw University in Raleigh, North Carolina.[15] Over the course of its existence, the medical school trained over 400 Black doctors, who performed well on state board exams and had successful practices in their local communities. In spite of the medical school's success, Shaw University reduced Leonard to a two-year program in 1914 and closed it in 1918.[16] Part of the problem for Leonard Medical School was a lack of money; without a substantial endowment and with few donations from Northern philanthropists and successful alumni, the institution was bound to fail.[17]

White-led missionary groups established the medical department at Knoxville College in Knoxville, Tennessee, in 1895 and Flint Medical School in New Orleans, Louisiana, in 1899.[18] A medical department established in 1870 for Blacks in the North, at Pennsylvania's Lincoln University, lasted only six years. Because of its remote location, nearly 30 miles from Philadelphia, and a lack of financial support, Lincoln could not afford to maintain the program. Over the course of its existence, Lincoln University's medical department produced only six graduates.[19]

A few Black doctors who were graduates of these early programs opened their own proprietary medical schools, just as many White doctors were doing.[20] These Black schools included Louisville National Medical College (1888), Hannibal Medical College (1889), Chattanooga National Medical College (1889), Knoxville Medical College (1900), and the University of West Tennessee College of Medicine and Surgery (1907).[21] Unlike their missionary-sponsored counterparts, which were affiliated with colleges and universities, Black proprietary medical schools did not have an institution to fall back on in times of need.[22] Not only did they lack buildings, libraries, and other campus resources, but they were less appealing to students' parents in another way. According to Savitt, at college- and university-sponsored medical schools, "students were able to live and study in the controlled setting of a college environment, a feature that parents, especially those from rural areas who were distrustful of the supposed bad influences of cities and concerned about their children's safety, liked."[23] Parents, in particular, were grateful that missionary schools combined moral and religious education with medical school education.

Although most medical publications reported on the successes and the needs of mainstream Black medical schools, proprietary schools received no coverage.[24] Similarly, funders such as the Slater Fund, the Carnegie Foundation, and the Rockefeller-sponsored General Education Board ignored the proprietary schools, focusing on missionary-sponsored institutions instead.[25] And some proprietary schools, both Black and White, were basically diploma mills; the reputation of the legitimate proprietary schools suffered as a result. Most funders lumped all proprietary schools into the same negative category.

Proprietary schools in general, regardless of racial makeup, provided medical services to poorer communities; they also offered opportunities for poor young people to enter the medical profession. A credential from one of these institutions, however, was not wholly respected in either the Black or the White community.[26] By 1920, Black proprietary schools had fallen by the wayside, unable to keep up with their university-sponsored counterparts.[27] They were also hamstrung by a lack of confidence (often justified) on the part of the public. Black medical schools in general faced an extra obstacle, as many Whites in the medical profession doubted the ability of these graduates to pass the licensing exam.[28] Regardless of type, all Black medical institutions would soon confront a nearly insurmountable struggle as the quest for uniform standards in medical education emerged.

The Introduction of Standards

In 1904 the American Medical Association established the Council on Medical Education, which began promoting higher standards in medical education. These included a minimum standard for physicians, "calling for four years of high school, an equal period of medical training, and passage of a licensing test."[29] The council also began grading medical schools on their graduates' success on state licensing examinations, eventually extending its evaluations to medical school curricula, facilities, admissions requirements, and faculty.[30] According to Savitt, the council's actions, though directed at all medical schools and not Black schools in particular, "put these [latter] institutions on notice."[31] Many Black colleges complied with the council's policies and recommendations, "lengthening their terms, improving hospital and laboratory facilities, and, at least in written documents, toughening entrance and graduation requirements."[32] Black medical school leaders knew that they would need to make changes to survive in an increasingly technologically advanced society. But before long another layer of requirements and standards would appear that were too stringent for most of these institutions to meet.[33]

The Flexner Report

Abraham Flexner graduated from the Johns Hopkins University in 1886 at the age of 19. After teaching briefly at his high school in Louisville, Kentucky, he established a college preparatory school there to test his ideas about how inspired teaching could help youth succeed. In 1905 he pursued graduate work in education at Harvard University, where he nurtured his interest in graduate and professional education. Flexner published his first book, *The American College*, in 1908. The young scholar was deeply critical of American higher education and especially of the university lecture as a method of instruction. He preferred small classes with hands-on instruction, believing that students responded to enthusiastic teaching and were hampered by the rules and regulations that schools placed on them.[34]

Flexner's book attracted the attention of Henry Pritchett, the president of the Carnegie Foundation for the Advancement of Teaching. Pritchett was

TABLE I.I
Black Medical Schools Evaluated by Flexner, 1908–1910
(1,253 total graduates from inception to Flexner inspection)

Institution	Location	Number of graduates	Dates of operation
Howard University Medical College	Washington, DC	205	1868–present
Knoxville Medical College	Knoxville, TN	2	1900–1910
Leonard Medical School, Shaw University	Raleigh, NC	400	1882–1918
Louisville National Medical College	Louisville, KY	100	1888–1912
Meharry Medical College	Nashville, TN	275	1876–present
New Orleans University Medical College (Flint Medical College)	New Orleans, LA	116	1889–1911
University of West Tennessee College of Physicians and Surgeons	Jackson, TN	155	1900–1923

Sources: Data from Louis W. Sullivan and Ilana Suez Mittman, "The State of Diversity in the Health Professions a Century after Flexner," *Academic Medicine*, vol. 85, no. 2 (Feb. 2010), 247. See also Earl H. Harley, "The Forgotten History of Defunct Black Medical Schools in the 19th and 20th Centuries and the Impact of the Flexner Report," *Journal of the National Medical Association*, vol. 98, no. 9 (2006), 1425–1429.

looking for someone to lead a series of evaluations of professional education. Although Flexner had never studied medicine or visited a medical school, he was Pritchett's top choice to lead an examination of American medical education, based on his educational background and his interest in critiquing American higher education.[35] Flexner joined the research staff at the Carnegie Foundation in 1908; in 1910, working on behalf of the foundation and the American Medical Association, he issued a report on the state of American medical education that led to vast reforms in the way doctors were trained.

According to Flexner, the model medical school, in terms of curriculum and pedagogy, was Johns Hopkins.[36] He wanted to see all American medical schools adopt its model, which included, among other things, a four-year program and an admissions requirement of a high school diploma and two years of college.[37] The Flexner report, based on visits to 155 medical schools in the United States and Canada, led to the closing of most rural medical schools, proprietary schools, and all but two of the nation's seven Black medical colleges (table 1.1).[38]

Though Blacks made up only 10.6 percent of the nation's citizens at the time of the Flexner report, they were by far the largest racial or ethnic minority.[39] Blacks had a shorter average life expectancy than did Whites: for Black women, life expectancy was 35 years, and for Black men, a mere 32. In comparison, average life expectancy for Whites was 48 years for males and 51 years for females.[40] Diseases such as tuberculosis and typhoid fever, as well as inadequate medical facilities and dire poverty, contributed to the infant mortality rate and early deaths of many Blacks. They were in desperate need of doctors and increased access to health care. But Flexner argued that Black medical schools did little to alleviate the health problems of Blacks, and that they were "wasting small sums annually and sending out undisciplined men, whose lack of real training is covered up by the imposing M.D. degree."[41]

Although they tried to adapt to increasingly stringent standards, Black medical schools had little capacity for large-scale change. The proprietary schools had only student tuition and the occasional small, local investor as sources of income. Philanthropists were not interested in giving their money or support to what seemed to them to be diploma mills. Though missionary-sponsored schools had slightly more access to capital, in reality their finances were still precarious. Because Black college students, for the most part, came from poor families that had immense difficulty paying tuition and fees, Black medical schools could expect scant funds from them.[42] Having no steady source of income meant that the schools had to skimp, making it difficult to offer a robust program.

Flexner's report, which dedicated only a few pages to Black medical schools, called for the closure of five of the remaining seven institutions (at a high point there had been 14 of them). Flexner found Meharry and Howard medical schools to be acceptable. These two institutions would be left to educate enough doctors to serve a population of 12 million Blacks in a segregated society at the beginning of the twentieth century. And even these two institutions were almost forced to close.[43] According to Paul Starr, the limited number of Black medical schools had a substantial impact for years to come. Even 20 years after the Flexner report, Blacks were still severely circumscribed, with only one Black doctor for every 3,000 African Americans. In the South, the situation was much direr. For example, in Mississippi there was one Black doctor for every 14,634 Black people.[44]

Flexner respected George W. Hubbard, the founder of Meharry Medical School. He admired Hubbard's ability to stretch scarce resources and build an institution with the proper facilities.[45] And Howard, with its annual federal appropriation and clinical privileges at the Freedmen's Hospital, had what Flexner saw as guaranteed stability.[46] Interestingly, when Flexner critiqued the Black medical schools, he also made funding recommendations, urging philanthropists to support only Meharry and Howard, thus starving the other schools.[47] Flexner worked hand in hand with both the Carnegie and Rockefeller foundations, and they valued his opinion.[48] For example, the Rockefeller-sponsored General Education Board contributed substantially to schools to educate African Americans that were recommended by Flexner.[49] Nonetheless, according to Savitt, most Black medical schools were "caught in a power squeeze between two large foundations that put white medical education needs above black, and a powerful medical organization that refused to recognize the special needs of African American medical schools and African American physicians."[50]

That powerful medical organization was the AMA, which, at the time, was not interested in including African Americans among its membership.[51] To be a member of the AMA, a doctor also had to be a member of his or her state medical organization. Of course, in the South it was next to impossible for an African American to gain membership in a state chapter. Instead of the AMA, Black doctors and medical schools had their own organization, the National Medical Association (NMA).[52] The NMA was founded by African American doctors in 1896, after the Cotton States Exposition in Atlanta—an event intended to promote the Southern region and its products and manpower to the world as well as to increase trade. In reaction to the exclusion of African American doctors by many state and local medical societies in the midst of the South's celebration of its innovations, a new organization was born.[53] According to one scholar: "This peculiar duplication reflected a profession segregated by race. The AMA was almost entirely white; the NMA predominantly black." This professional segregation lasted well into the civil rights era.[54]

Not only were Blacks excluded from the mainstream medical establishment, but that establishment held a condescending view of their role and ability in the practice of medicine. Flexner's report exemplified this and "prescribed a limited role for black physicians in their practices and hinted that black physicians possessed less potential and ability than their white counterparts."[55] Some of the views Flexner expressed were clearly racist, such as the idea that Black doctors would never have enough skill to take care of White patients; Flexner said that "the practice of the Negro doctor will be limited to his own race."[56] Moreover, Flexner stated that the main reason to educate Black doctors was to serve the interests of the White race by stopping the spread of diseases from Blacks to Whites.[57] One article, in quoting Flexner's words, noted that he believed "Black physicians should be trained differently; namely, to 'humbly' serve 'their people' as 'sanitarians.' "[58] While Flexner was willing to grant that medical schools should educate men and women together, he was not nearly as progressive when it came to race. His report strengthened segregated and unequal medical education for African Americans.[59]

African Americans Practicing Medicine

In the early twentieth century, Meharry and Howard medical schools together produced more than 100 graduates annually.[60] However, even this small number could not find suitable internships in a segregated society. Only a few African Americans, less than 10 a year, graduated from the nation's other medical colleges. The vast majority of schools accepted no Blacks. Beginning in the 1930s, some Southern states provided out-of-state scholarships to Black citizens wanting to attend graduate school, including medical school—but only as a way to prevent these individuals from attending in-state graduate programs.[61] The limited production of Black doctors was a significant problem for the African American community.[62]

By the 1940s, the number of Black physicians was growing. But access to quality health care, or health care at all for that matter, was still limited for most Blacks. The ratio of Black physicians to Blacks in general continued to be very low and grew even more so as the decade progressed. In the Southern states in 1942, for example, historian Joseph Johnson noted that there was one White physician for every 1,060 White citizens and one Black physician for every 5,832 Black citizens.[63] By 1948, the situation had worsened: there was one White doctor for every 1,262 White citizens and one Black doctor for every 6,203 Black citizens. The state of Georgia, in particular, had a dire situation, with one Black doctor for every 7,134 Black citizens in 1942 and one Black doctor for every 7,384 Black citizens in 1948. Johnson attributes the decline in physicians of both races to the call-up of doctors for service in the military in World War II.

Compounding the shortage of Black doctors was the low enrollment of African Americans in medical school, in part because of discrimination in admissions policies and in society at large. For instance, in 13 of the Southern states (Alabama, Arkansas, Florida, Georgia, Kentucky, Louisiana, Mississippi, North Carolina, Oklahoma, South Carolina, Tennessee, Texas, and Virginia), only 234 Blacks were enrolled in medical school in 1948, all of them at Meharry Medical College in Tennessee. In the border states of Delaware, Maryland, and West Virginia, as well as in the District of Columbia, there were only 267 Black medical students—all of them at Howard University.

Medical schools in the rest of the country enrolled a few African Americans, most of them in New York (23), Michigan (17), and Pennsylvania (10).[64] Moreover, in 1948, out of a total of 80 U.S. medical schools, the 26 located in the South and Border States had policies that expressly prohibited the enrollment of African Americans.[65] As late as 1964, five Southern medical schools *still* had policies that prohibited the admission of Blacks.[66] These included the Medical College of Alabama, the Medical College of Georgia, Louisiana State University School of Medicine, the University of Mississippi School of Medicine, and the Medical College of South Carolina.[67]

One of the most difficult aspects of medical training for African Americans was obtaining a residency after graduation.[68] A residency allows new physicians to enhance their clinical skills and hone their knowledge of a specialty.[69] Racial discrimination was the main reason that few Black doctors were able to secure residencies between 1896 and 1965. White hospitals and universities did not want to employ them, for fear that patients would complain and also because many White doctors refused to work alongside Blacks as equals.[70] Often, Black doctors, regardless of their credentials, would be given "scut work" or the tasks no one else wanted to do in hospitals.[71] Some Black doctors, ever resourceful, would gain clinical skills at small, rural hospitals where medical help was desperately needed. Because of intense discrimination in the specialties, most Black doctors became general practitioners or family practitioners, starting a long history of the commitment of African American physicians to primary care. A few courageous Black doctors pursued specialties in obstetrics, gynecology, or pediatrics, but they struggled to set up successful practices amid the racial bias of the times.[72] According to Wilbur Watson, "the more technical specialties, such as pathology, ophthalmology, physical medicine and rehabilitation, and surgery did not begin to show up in substantial numbers among the ranks of African American physicians until after the *Brown v. Board of Education* decision of 1954 and the amended Hill-Burton Act of 1965."[73] Once it was amended to drop a "separate but equal" clause, the Hill-Burton Act required hospitals and other social service institutions that received federal funds to provide services to everyone in their surrounding communities, regardless of color, race, country of origin, creed, or the ability to speak English.[74] The passage of the Civil Rights Act of 1964 and the creation of Medicare in 1965 also played a part in desegregating the nation's hospitals, thus making medicine a more feasible and desirable career goal for young African Americans.[75]

Federal support of civil rights helped open the doors of some segregated universities to African American medical students. For instance, in 1963 Delano Meriwether was admitted to Duke University's medical school, Hamilton Holmes was accepted at Emory University's medical school that year after the Georgia Supreme Court ruled that private institutions could accept Blacks, and Levi Watkins Jr. enrolled at Vanderbilt University's medical school in 1966—the last three Southern medical schools with all-white student bodies.[76] And in the late 1960s, federally backed affirmative action programs became more common at many historically White medical schools. As a result, from 1969 to 1974 the yearly number of African American medical school graduates rose from 153 to 571—about a sixfold increase in graduates from the late 1940s.[77] By 1998, the 1,211 Black medical school graduates accounted for 7.5 percent of all physicians graduating in the United States.[78] But even the 1998 numbers were not proportionate: 7.5 percent of graduating physicians from a group that represented about 13 percent of the overall population. As these figures suggest, historically White medical schools in the South and throughout the country have not produced a sufficient number of Black doctors.[79] The medical schools that have graduated the most Black physicians since 1950 are listed in table 1.2. Only one of them is a historically White institution in the South.

Despite an increased presence of Blacks in medical schools throughout the country in recent years, there have been gender disparities among the African Americans who have attended them. Over the past half century, over 25,000 African Americans have graduated from medical school and, of these graduates, 59 percent have been men.[80] As late as 1972, for instance, African American men made up 86 percent of all Black medical school graduates. More recently, however, the situation has greatly changed. Starting in 1989 and in every subsequent year, African American women have accounted for the majority of graduates from Black medical schools.[81]

The Origin of an Idea

Given the pervasive discrimination against Blacks in the medical profession and in the provision of medical care, it is not surprising that African Americans have sought over the years to create their own medical schools. But fashioning a medical school from the ground up is easier said than done. As mentioned earlier, of the 47 new medical schools begun during the second half of the twentieth century, Morehouse School of Medicine is the only four-year, accredited medical school whose student body is predominantly Black.

TABLE I.2

Medical Schools Producing the Most Black Graduates, 1950–2010

Medical school	Number of Black graduates	Year founded
Howard University	3,671	1868
Meharry Medical College	3,032	1876
University of Illinois	580	1913
Wayne State University	568	1868
University of Michigan	473	1850
Temple University	446	1901
Harvard University	431	1782
University of Medicine and Dentistry of New Jersey	410	1954
University of North Carolina	408	1879
SUNY-Brooklyn	391	1860
Case Western Reserve University	352	1843
SUNY-Buffalo	335	1850
Morehouse School of Medicine	314	1975

Sources: Association of American Medical Colleges, Annual Status of Medical Education report, 2010, Morehouse School of Medicine Archives; "Naming Selective Colleges That Are Most Preferred by Black Students," *Journal of Blacks in Higher Education*, vol. 30 (Winter 2000/2001), 28.

Note: Morehouse School of Medicine has only been in existence since 1975 and has graduated a mere 300 fewer students than the top-producing historically White institutions over the past 50 years. Interestingly, the University of Michigan has a track record stretching back to the mid-1930s in terms of admitting Black medical students. Starting in roughly 1935, that institution admitted about 10 Black students a year—outside of Howard University and Meharry Medical College, this is more than any single medical school. See Joseph L. Johnson, "The Supply of Negro Health Personnel—Physicians," *Journal of Negro Education*, vol. 18, no. 3 (Summer 1949), 346–356.

Interestingly, in 1906 John Hope, the first African American president of Morehouse College, proposed a medical school near Atlanta's other Black colleges. He sought to merge the five Black colleges into one strong university with undergraduate, graduate, and professional schools; eventually, this idea led to the creation of a consortium among three of the colleges in 1929, as the Atlanta University Center Affiliation. This later evolved into a collaborative effort among all of the Black colleges in the historic West End District of Atlanta. These institutions together occupy over 200 acres of land. Each college is independent, with its own students, board of trustees, president, faculty, and staff. Because the institutions had different religious affiliations and academic cultures, it was not possible to merge them into a single institution, as Hope desired.[82]

To pursue his idea of a medical school, in 1922 Hope recruited a Black physician from Chicago, Marque Jackson, an alumnus of Morehouse College. But in 1929 the Great Depression hit, and the Black community was disproportionately affected. As a result, Hope told Jackson that the development of a medical school would have to wait for better economic times.[83] Physician Asa G. Yancey Sr., interviewed at age 96 in May 2008, remembered hearing about the medical school idea: "I've heard since I was a little boy—5, 6, 7, 10 years old—that the medical school should be developed in Atlanta, and be associated with the Atlanta University colleges. That's something that was mentioned at intervals all throughout my childhood."[84] But after John Hope died in 1933, the idea of a medical school at the Atlanta University Center lay dormant until the 1960s.[85]

CHAPTER TWO

Birth of a Medical School

The Medical Education Program at Morehouse College was born in the midst of racial turmoil and during a time of limited opportunity for African American students and Black physicians. A key factor in its birth was a 1967 report, *Physician Manpower in Georgia*, released by the Georgia Office of Comprehensive Health Planning, which warned that the state was facing a dire shortage of medical doctors. According to this document, Georgia's population, which stood at about 4.6 million and was growing faster than that of the nation as a whole, was expected to reach almost 5 million people by 1975.[1] Increases in the population, according to the report, would certainly call for greater numbers of health care professionals. However, Georgia ranked at number 38 among the 50 states in terms of physician manpower per capita.[2]

In the late 1960s and early 1970s, there was a shortage of physicians across the nation. This shortage had been projected in 1959 by the Bane Report to the Surgeon General of the United States,[3] which noted that "the problem of the growing need for physicians for this country stems from a combination of three major phenomena: the rapid growth of the population; the increase in the use of personal medical services; and the increase in the number of physicians required for specialized services."[4] Even to maintain the present physician-population ratio, the report said, the anticipated 1975 U.S. population of 235 million would require 330,000 doctors. This number necessitated the yearly graduation of 11,000 medical students—an increase of approximately 3,600 over the number in 1959.[5] Of particular importance to the idea of a new medical school in Atlanta was the report's call for the expansion of medical schools.[6]

As a result of these projected national trends, states were intensifying their efforts to increase the number of doctors.[7] At the end of 1968, only 1.67 percent of practicing doctors were Black, while the nation's population was approximately 11 percent Black.[8] According to one study, "if the ratio of Black population to Black physicians was equal to the United States' White population to White physicians' ratio (560 persons per physician), an additional 35,000 Black physicians would have been required in 1968."[9] When considering Southeastern states, including Alabama, Georgia, Florida, Mississippi,

TABLE 2.1
Distribution of Black Physicians by State, 1968

State	Number of Black physicians	Population of state
Alabama	61	3,446,000
California	574	19,394,000
District of Columbia	417	778,000
Florida	82	6,433,000
Georgia	95	4,482,000
Illinois	265	10,995,000
Louisiana	62	3,603,000
Massachusetts	43	5,618,000
Michigan	0	8,696,000
Minnesota	19	3,703,000
Mississippi	44	2,219,000
New York	562	18,051,000
Tennessee	133	3,878,000
Texas	135	10,819,000

Sources: Asa G. Yancey Sr., "Negroes in Medicine: A Surgeon Looks at Leaders in the Years of Black Emergence in American Medicine," *Medicine at Emory*, vol. 8 (1970), 12–18. See also Bureau of the Census, U.S. Department of Commerce, "Intercensal Estimates of the Total Resident Population of States: 1960 to 1970," www.census.gov/popest/archives/1980s/st6070ts.txt.

North Carolina, South Carolina, and Tennessee, there would have been a need for approximately 12,000 additional Black physicians to achieve a comparable Black population to Black physician ratio.[10] The problem was nationwide, as shown in table 2.1. An important statistic is that the number of Black physicians was lower in states with higher Black populations.

In Georgia specifically, there were 795 White people for every White doctor but 13,810 Black people for every Black doctor.[11] According to the *Medical Directory of Georgia*, in 1970 there were 3,927 practicing physicians in Georgia, of whom only 95 were Black.[12] These disparities contributed to enormous health issues across the state. Although segregation had been outlawed across the nation, it was still the practice in many Southern states for Black patients to be served almost exclusively by Black doctors.[13] Many studies found an urgent need to increase the number of Black students pursuing a medical career; only one in 20 Georgia students entering medical school in the late 1960s was Black.[14] Between 1963 and 1969, the two medical schools in Georgia together graduated only one Black doctor. By 1970, Emory University and the Medical College of Georgia enrolled only 23 Black students. This figure was a substantial increase over the previous 10 years, but given the vast need in the South for Black doctors, much more would have to be done.[15]

A report titled *Medical School Alumni of 1967* showed that 57 percent of Black MD students from Georgia who graduated from Meharry and Howard returned to Georgia to practice.[16] It is worth mentioning that these two medical schools were constantly under the microscope and periodically teetered on the edge of closing. In 1968, sociologists Christopher Jencks and David Riesman referred to them as "the worst in the nation" and claimed that they "would probably have been closed long ago had they not been a main source of doctors willing to tend Negro patients."[17]

According to the 1967 *Physician Manpower* report, Black physicians in Georgia were aging and few young people were replacing them.[18] The average age of a Black physician in Georgia was 54, compared with 43 for White physicians. The report estimated that by 1980, roughly 40 percent of Georgia's Black physicians would have reached age 70, died, or retired. Moreover, the report noted that the health of Georgians was below the national average, and that access to primary care was a significant problem for the state's citizens. According to Paul Starr, although the 1960s witnessed a rise in the use of medical services by the poor, most of these gains were in the North rather than the South.[19]

National data in 1970 showed that 83 percent of the nation's Black physicians had graduated from Meharry Medical College or Howard University College of Medicine.[20] Other medical schools in the United States graduated only 15 percent of these MDs; the remaining 2 percent of the nation's Black doctors earned their degrees abroad. Most of those other U.S. schools were in the Midwest—schools such as the University of Michigan and the University of Illinois.[21] In 1968, Meharry and Howard graduated 144 Black physicians, while the other 99 medical schools in the nation graduated a total of 56 Black doctors.[22] There was an obvious need for another Black medical school, especially in the South, as the majority of Black doctors were practicing in California, New York, and Washington, D.C.[23]

A "Crazy" Idea for Atlanta University

A year after *Physician Manpower in Georgia* came out, Louis Brown, an African American physician who practiced internal medicine in Atlanta, brought the idea for a new medical school to the presidents of the schools in the Atlanta University Center. Brown was the cochair of the committee that issued the report. The committee also recommended that Georgia have more than its two current medical schools (Emory University's School of Medicine and the Medical College of Georgia). They suggested expanding medical education so that more of the state's young people could train in Georgia and would

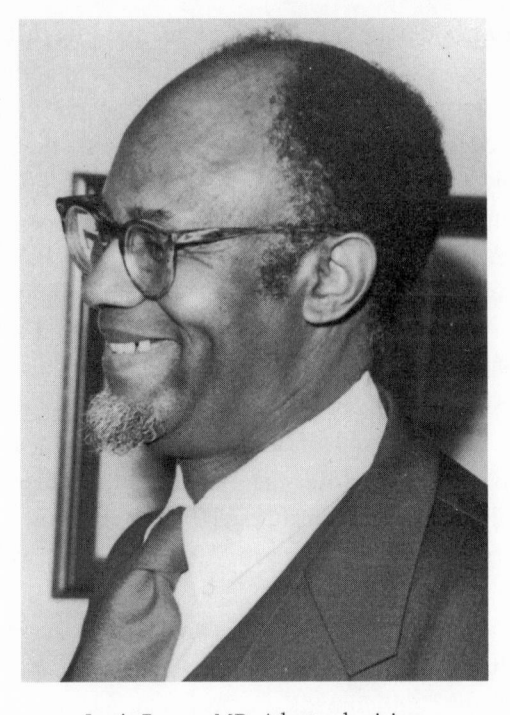

Louis Brown, MD, Atlanta physician.

stay in the state after receiving their medical degrees.[24] Inspired by the possibilities, Brown got on the agenda of the Atlanta University Center presidents' monthly meeting. He argued that the report justified developing another Black medical school.[25] Brown pointed out that there was a shortage of Black physicians across the country and certainly in Georgia. He also argued that the Atlanta University Center was the most logical place for a third predominantly Black medical school. Brown said that the combination of the academic environment, the size and the financial strengths of the Center, and its location in the growing economic environment of Atlanta made this location much more sensible than Birmingham, Alabama, or Charlotte, North Carolina.[26]

At first the Atlanta University Center presidents thought Brown's idea was little more than fantasy.[27] According to Clinton Warner, a future board chair of Morehouse School of Medicine, "when Louie Brown told Tom Jarrett, the president of Atlanta University, Jarrett almost laughed in his face."[28] Eventually, however, Brown convinced Jarrett and others to do a feasibility study.

From its conception, the idea of the medical school received support not only from Georgia's Black physicians (Louis Brown was president of the Georgia State Medical Association, the state chapter of the National Medical Association), but from many White physicians as well. This was due to the influence of the other cochair of the manpower committee, Rhodes Haverty, who was president of the Medical Association of Georgia, the state chapter of the American Medical Association.[29] Brown and Haverty worked together to gain the support of both Black and White physicians in the state.[30] The idea of a medical school affiliated with the Atlanta University Center represented a coming together of the AMA and the NMA, and it was evidence that the Georgia AMA was changing—its members were willing to shed their discriminatory past and move forward in support of African American medical education.

In November 1968, Atlanta University's Board of Trustees authorized the president and faculty to investigate the idea.[31] President Jarrett convened a committee of faculty to initiate the study; early in the process, he invited the dean and faculty of Emory University's School of Medicine to contribute their thoughts. After quite a bit of work, the Board of Trustees voted in 1969 to proceed with the feasibility study. But Atlanta University did not have enough funds to support a full feasibility study, and it had to solicit money from foundations. The Josiah Macy Jr. Foundation was a main contributor to the effort, providing $21,500.[32]

Before engaging in the full-blown feasibility study, Jarrett worked to gauge the attitudes and opinions of the local community. He discussed the idea with his faculty and with the presidents of the Atlanta University Center schools (Spelman College, Morehouse College, Clark College, and Morris Brown College), he talked with the Black doctors who were members of the Atlanta Medical Association, and he engaged prominent alumni in a conversation to garner their support.[33] With the help of Bernard Hallman, an associate dean of the medical school at Emory University, Jarrett also brought together the top administrators of five medical schools and organizations to help him think through the idea. On January 14 and 15, 1971, the leaders of Dartmouth Medical School, Meharry Medical College, Stanford University School of Medicine, and the Veterans Administration Medical Services, as well as the Association of American Medical Colleges' president, John A. D. Cooper, met to analyze Atlanta University's potential for establishing a new medical school to serve Blacks in the region.[34] Emory University paid the expenses of everyone who attended the meeting.[35] The leaders of Meharry and the Veterans Administration had experience working with African

American medical students and patients, but those at elite institutions such as Dartmouth and Stanford did not. Although the input of these latter two individuals was valuable, their perspective was quite different. They were operating with considerably more resources and a set of goals for medical education that did not focus on primary care and serving the underserved.[36]

At last the feasibility study was carried out. At Jarrett's request, Fry Consultants Inc. studied the possibility of adding a two-year basic medical school to Atlanta University.[37] The consultants considered whether the medical school could eventually be merged into a four-year program, the availability of qualified faculty members, sources of funding to sustain operations, physical plant needs, the needs of the region, and the attitude toward the idea in both the city of Atlanta and the state of Georgia.[38]

The consultants confirmed the need for a new medical school aimed at training Black doctors. But they were uncertain that Atlanta University could afford such a venture. They advised that Atlanta University would need to design an appropriate curriculum, acquire adequate staffing, establish a close relationship with Emory University and other medical schools, and have enough capital to build first-rate facilities, cover continuing operations, and purchase land for the school's growth.[39] Based on their investigation of medical school curricula throughout the country, Fry Consultants asserted that if Atlanta University were to establish a medical school, it would have to "rapidly develop into a four-year school." In the interim, the institution would have to create linkages with four-year programs to ensure a smooth transfer for students entering their third year.[40]

One of the main concerns Fry expressed was that Atlanta University would find it hard to attract faculty to the new medical school. They said that it would be hard to draw professors to the institution because it would lack the reputation and prestige of an established medical school, would not have comparable research facilities and equipment, and might face a stigma for being a "Black" institution. Its location in the Deep South would be also a liability, because many professors held negative views of the region.[41] According to the consultants, Atlanta University's ability to establish and maintain a medical school would depend completely on Emory University. The institution would need to establish a third-year transfer program with Emory, and it would need to ask for help from Emory's faculty as well as its accreditation and fundraising mechanisms. It would also need to use Emory's equipment and research facilities.[42] All of these aspects of the partnership with Emory had been discussed in 1968, when President Jarrett met with Bernard Hall-man, the associate dean at Emory's School of Medicine.[43]

In previous decades, most medical schools had shifted their mission, plac-ing a greater emphasis on research because of the prestige and funding it brings to an institution.[44] But an emphasis on research means additions to the physical plant of a campus. Fry consultants said that several new build-ings and additional land would be needed in order for Atlanta University to host a medical school, in order to accommodate faculty members' research and teaching as well as to provide student housing. Although the nation's medical schools typically received a substantial portion of their funding from the federal government—in 1970, roughly 43 percent—Fry estimated that this type of funding was decreasing and would become harder to obtain.[45] According to Paul Starr, there was ample medical funding during the John-son administration, as part of the Great Society programs aimed at improv-ing the quality of life for Americans overall. The 1970s, however, ushered in an era of doubt among public officials, including both President Nixon and the Democratic Congress. They "began to regard the aggregate costs of health care as too high and to doubt that the investment was worth the return in health."[46]

Although colleges and universities saw the reauthorization of the Higher Education Act in 1972, medical schools were not hopeful in terms of in-creased funding from the federal government.[47] Private medical schools had an especially hard time acquiring funds. Nonetheless, Fry Consultants noted that a new medical school for Blacks might appeal to the government because of the national need for Black physicians. Moreover, President Nixon had made some overtures to African Americans during his presidency. For ex-ample, he had created the National Biomedical Science Research Program, which was aimed at sending more minorities into the biomedical sciences. This program provided grants to colleges and universities. Nixon also created the National Sickle Cell Program, which targeted a disease that affects Blacks almost exclusively.[48] In addition to federal funding, Fry Consultants estimated that a new medical school could attract money from some private foundations but noted that this type of funding was limited.[49]

According to Fry, the most serious obstacle Atlanta University faced was financial.[50] Adding a medical school to the existing institution would have cost roughly $29 million, and the maximum expected income from it would be approximately $10 million short, thus making it necessary for Atlanta

University to raise a substantial amount of money. The consultants were concerned that the university could not solicit this much for a number of reasons, including a feeling among Whites in Atlanta that "out-of-towners" had supported the institution in the past and should continue to do so. At one time, beginning during Reconstruction, Northern White philanthropic activities in the South were closely tied to the industrial interests of the philanthropists who supported them. White Southerners' self-justification of their racist attitudes was tied to quite real fears that these Northerners were exploiting them. Thus Southern Whites had often claimed that their antagonism toward Black equality was an antagonism toward outsiders trying to "change their way of life." Southern Whites often believed that the liberal arts–focused Black colleges, like those in the Atlanta University Center, were creating a class of "uppity Negroes."[51] Black colleges, especially liberal arts ones, had a long history of being supported by Whites from the North—be they missionaries or industrial philanthropists. The Rockefellers, for example, supported Spelman College, and the institution was named after John D. Rockefeller's wife.[52] Even Southerners who were more liberal had given little money to these institutions; thus there was concern that Whites in Atlanta and Georgia would not be willing to fund a new medical school.[53]

After meeting with leaders at Atlanta University, interviewing various constituents in Atlanta and Georgia, reviewing statistical information on the medical profession, and examining the potential operating costs, the consulting firm determined that although there was sufficient need for a new medical school, they would recommend against its establishment for lack of finances:

> It is extremely questionable whether Atlanta University could obtain enough firm financial commitments to adequately support the school. Atlanta University itself could not supply large amounts of money to the program. In the view of recent cutbacks in federal spending and lack of increase in foundation support, there does not appear to be sufficient basis of continuing financial support from other sources. Unless the federal government provides the great majority of the required funding through existing or specially designed programs, the proposed school of basic medical sciences at Atlanta University will not be realized.[54]

The external consultants from prestigious medical schools convened by Emory University agreed. They held that "Atlanta University should not attempt such a program at the present time." They made the recommendation with deep regret: "We all recognized the need for a greater output of physicians from the State of Georgia and a particular need for Black physicians. These are, however, extremely difficult times for medical schools, and the financial problems associated with the development of such an institution mitigate against implementation at this time."[55]

Interestingly, several of the early proponents of the medical school believed that President Jarrett commissioned a feasibility study merely to avoid criticism from the Black community.[56] Jarrett was an English professor rooted in the humanities, and some felt that he was not fully committed to the idea of a medical school; others even thought that he stacked the committee to get a recommendation to cease moving forward.[57] Institutional lore recalls that Jarrett was warned by a number of people that medical schools were a lot of trouble. He was told that they were expensive, had faculties with big egos who wanted big salaries, and required a lot of laboratory space.[58]

Hugh Gloster Steps Up to the Plate

When the vote not to proceed with the medical school idea passed at the Atlanta University trustees meeting in April 1971, Morehouse College president Hugh Gloster stood up and said, "Well, now that you have voted, let me ask if there would be any objection by Atlanta University to Morehouse College looking at this question, because we have an interest here." Gloster had an advantage over Atlanta University in starting a medical school—Morehouse College already had a strong premedical program.[59] Year after year, out of this Black college's graduating class of roughly 60 students, 20 students on average pursued medical and dental degrees or PhDs in the sciences.[60] According to data from the Association of American Medical Colleges, when Gloster raised the idea of Morehouse College starting a medical school, the college was the second largest producer of African Americans pursuing medical degrees, after Howard University.[61]

Gloster had been investigating the medical school idea behind the scenes. He had asked for the assistance of William Bennett, a new employee of the National Institutes of Health's (NIH) Bureau of Manpower, which was responsible for supporting new medical schools.[62] Bennett, who did not realize at first that Gloster was interested in the medical school idea, was actually relieved when Atlanta University decided not to pursue it. He noted that "very few schools have that kind of money, those kinds of resources. I was happy that Atlanta University had the good sense to pass on the idea."[63] According to Bennett, when Gloster "stood up, walked to the front and said, 'My Board of Trustees has authorized me to report that we are prepared to develop a

medical school if the Board of Trustees of Atlanta University decides not to,'
I said, 'This man is crazy; he's got no sense at all.' "[64]

None of the Atlanta University trustees objected to Gloster's interest, although most thought it was a far-fetched idea and would never be realized.[65]
But Gloster saw the possibilities, especially in terms of educating African
American doctors who focused on primary care in urban and rural communities. Although the Morehouse president was a staunch proponent of integration and thought that predominantly White medical schools should work
diligently to enroll African Americans, he also understood that Blacks needed
institutions dedicated to their own growth and education. He learned this
while living as a Black man in the segregated South. Like other Black college
presidents navigating the waters of a legally desegregated yet still not equal
society, Gloster had to advocate simultaneously for integration and for continued support for Black colleges to ensure that African Americans were af-
forded educational opportunities. Immediately after the *Brown v. Board of
Education* decision, this type of maneuvering became the norm for Black college presidents, and some would argue that it still is.[66]

One obstacle for Morehouse College was that the bylaws of the Atlanta
University Center, established in 1929, assigned graduate and professional
education to Atlanta University (now Clark-Atlanta University) and undergraduate or baccalaureate instruction to the colleges. Technically, for one of
the colleges to initiate graduate or professional education was a violation of
the bylaws. The solution came when Atlanta University essentially granted
permission to Morehouse College to reach beyond the traditional role these
institutions had played.[67] On August 12, 1977, the Atlanta University Board
of Trustees passed a resolution stating:

> Since the feasibility study conducted by Fry Consultants, with respect to establish-
> ing a two-year medical school at Atlanta University . . . was not recommended, and
> since Atlanta University does not propose to develop a medical school, and does not
> see that it is feasible to do so, that the Atlanta University Board of Trustees wishes
> to make it clear that whichever way the two-year medical school at Morehouse Col-
> lege is developing, the University does not feel itself aggrieved.[68]

Knowing that Bill Bennett was at the meeting and was responsible for
working to support new medical schools throughout the nation under the
Carter administration,[69] after Gloster made his announcement and received
approval from the Atlanta University trustees to go forward with his idea, he
asked Bennett to come to the front of the room. Gloster asked Bennett

whether he would support Morehouse's medical school aspirations. In Bennett's words: "There was a hailstorm that started at almost that exact moment. I have no idea why, but I agreed to help Gloster and said I'd do everything in my power. It was eerie. I have never been able to explain it. I said I was going to help him [even though I was thinking], 'He can't develop a medical school.'"[70] After some reflection, Bennett followed up with Gloster, letting him know that "in addition to developing a need for a medical school, they had to develop the demand for a medical school."[71] Bennett asked him:

> Where are you going to get your students? Do you know the current enrollment in medical schools in the country? Do you know how many students are applying and not getting in? How many of those applying are qualified to be admitted and not getting in? What is the demand? And who's going to pay for this? Where are you going to get the faculty? Will White faculty be welcomed at Morehouse?[72]

All of these questions would need to be answered as Morehouse College moved forward with a medical school, but for now, the all-male Black college at least had Atlanta University's permission to pursue the idea.

Given Spelman College's reputation, one might wonder why it did not express interest in the medical school idea. In fact today, Spelman produces more Black women who enter graduate education in the sciences than any other college in the country, Black or White.[73] However, in the early to mid-1970s, Spelman did not have the same reputation in the sciences and pre-medical programs that Morehouse did. In addition, because of lack of opportunity and gender discrimination against all women, but especially Black women, the school had not been the alma mater of as many doctors as Morehouse had.[74] Moreover, Albert Manley, the president of Spelman at the time, had a rather patronizing view of women and their role in society.[75]

In spite of Atlanta University's initial green light for Morehouse, there were some objections to the all-male college pursuing a medical school. For example, at a meeting in November 1977 between the Executive Committees of the boards of trustees at Atlanta University and Morehouse College, Grace Hamilton, the vice-chair of Atlanta University's board and a prominent leader in the Atlanta Black community, objected on the grounds that Morehouse was a college and could not run a graduate program. President Hugh Gloster stood up and said:

> Recall that in April of 1971 at the board meeting I attended where Atlanta University trustees voted not to proceed with the medical school, I asked that since you de-

clined to create a medical school, would there be any objection to Morehouse College looking at this question and expressing our interest. There was no objection
raised. So it was on that basis that we proceeded with a number of things. We raised
funds for a feasibility study. Our plan for the medical school is not for Morehouse
College to operate this medical school indefinitely, but really to serve as the academic and administrative home for this new school until it has sufficiently developed to operate on its own.[76]

Gloster made it clear that the medical school would some day become independent of Morehouse College and would then have the option of applying
for membership in the Atlanta University Center.[77]

Nonetheless, Hamilton, who was also a Georgia legislator, tried to block
state funds from being distributed to Morehouse College for the medical
school. She believed that there was a "violation of the basic agreement regarding the cooperating institutions, with Atlanta University being designated for the graduate and professional education, with the exception of the
Interdenominational Theological Center."[78] Hamilton had personal reasons
for opposing the medical school—the Morehouse College president had fired
her husband, the college registrar, years earlier.[79] In spite of his opponents,
the persistent Black college leader pressed on, determined to prove that a
medical school at Morehouse College could have a profound impact.

Hamilton was not the only one who was less than happy with Gloster's
decision to move forward. On the copy of the medical school feasibility study
in the Atlanta University archives, someone wrote, "But Morehouse stole the
idea and proceeded with setting up the medical school"—an indication that
there may have been hard feelings about Gloster's efforts (the word "stole"
was crossed out and replaced with "took").[80] The Black colleges in the Atlanta
University Center cooperate in some instances and vie among themselves
in others.[81] For example, the Art Department at Spelman College serves as
the art department for all the schools in the Center, regardless of gender. On
the other hand, the schools compete with one another in athletics on the
same basis as they do with schools that are not affiliated with the Center.

Gloster persisted, despite any rivalries between the schools, and the idea
of a medical school at Morehouse would not have come to fruition without
his efforts. He was a highly successful president—named one of the nation's
best in 1986—and his college was considered top-notch as well. Gloster was
a Morehouse alumnus, and from the time he stepped into the role of president in 1967, he was deeply committed to the college's success and growth.

In the mid-1970s, Gloster launched a capital campaign for the school, bring-ing in more than $20 million, the most ever raised by a Black college at the time (though a small sum compared to more recent campaigns). Gloster also had to tackle the trouble that Black colleges were having in the 1970s in sus-taining enrollments during a time of increased integration.[82]

According to his wife, Yvonne, Hugh Gloster was an "aggressive man, with high energy, and was ahead of his time. He was so full of ideas that one almost had to tell him to slow down."[83] When Gloster decided to move for-ward with the medical school, many people at Morehouse and in the Black college community asked him why he would risk his legacy of successful leadership with such a bold plan for expansion.[84] He countered that it was the right time to expand the Morehouse campus in terms of both facilities and curriculum. In fact, he built 12 new buildings while president of Morehouse.[85] According to James Story, an alumnus of the college and the first faculty member of the Morehouse College medical program, Gloster's famed prede-cessor, President Benjamin Mays, was a builder of men, whereas Gloster was a builder of the campus. "All of the buildings that you see, Dr. Gloster did that. He couldn't replace Benjamin Mays; nobody could. But he seized the opportunity and created his own legacy for the institution."[86]

When he stepped down from the presidency of Morehouse College, Glos-ter felt that his greatest legacy was developing Morehouse School of Medi-cine.[87] In the words of longtime Morehouse supporter and physician Asa G. Yancey Sr., "Hugh Gloster threw the weight of Morehouse facilities and his strength and prestige behind it."[88]

Ready for Progress

During the late 1960s, according to Rhodes Haverty, "we were in a phase of American history where the doctor shortage was becoming more acute, and people were realizing that the best way of increasing the physician popula-tion of America and of Georgia was to increase the number of medical schools. There were only a few more than a hundred medical schools in the country at that time. One of the thoughts in Georgia was to establish another public medical school in Atlanta."[89] Atlanta was, and continues to be, the focal point of the state. It was the largest city and controlled much of the wealth, boasting the majority of the state's large corporations.[90]

The other question that people began to raise in the mid-1970s was related to the fight for integration taking place in higher education and in the nation as a whole. In the wake of all they had fought for during the civil rights struggles, many Black Americans found the idea of setting up an all-Black institution odd.[91] Morehouse College was arguing that the acute need for Black physicians would best be filled by a historically Black institution rather than an integrated, predominantly White institution. Ironically, the college's leadership also argued that its medical school would have an integrated faculty and student body.[92] Haverty was one person who understood this argument. He noted, "The push for integration was primarily, as I understand it, a push for equality in every aspect of life for Black people, and having their own medical school is one way to attain that."[93] He did not think that people thought of the Morehouse medical school as a step backward. Likewise, then governor Joe Frank Harris did not recall any objection at the state level to the establishment of a Black medical school. In his words, there was an attitude of "let's embrace the situation here"—the state had just recognized the Martin Luther King Jr. holiday, and attention was on how to eliminate the problems of the past rather than on generating new ones.[94]

Notably, the argument in support of a Black medical school in an era of integration was precisely the same as that used by Black colleges immediately after the *Brown v. Board of Education* decision. After 1954, Black college leaders made sure—without delay—that potential constituents, funders, and policymakers knew that these venerable institutions had never discriminated against or barred the admission of Whites. Now that legalized segregation had been dismantled, Black colleges would become diverse institutions, open to all, just like their historically White counterparts.[95] Of course, up to the present, very few historically Black or historically White institutions have fully integrated.

Morehouse School of Medicine, however—a Black institution established in an era of integration—had a firm commitment to the new order; over time, it has succeeded in attracting a diverse student body by offering a strong academic program. Interestingly, at both historically Black and historically White institutions, integration has always progressed more quickly at the graduate level than at the undergraduate level. At historically White institutions during the 1950s and 1960s, the integration of graduate programs seemed more acceptable to Whites. Perhaps the age of the students was a factor, especially in terms of the potential for men and women to mingle—a practice that was greatly feared in the South.[96] In addition, Southern states could not apply the principle of "separate but equal" to graduate programs, because there were no all-Black graduate programs in many fields. These states were, in fact, forced to integrate their graduate programs.[97] As mentioned previously, some Southern states sent African Americans out of state on scholarships to avoid educating them in the state, but others decided to admit Blacks. The NAACP Legal Defense Fund fought hard against segregation at the graduate level, because the establishment of separate graduate and professional schools was extremely costly. Between 1936 and 1950, the Legal Defense Fund fought, and won, several cases that made the out-of-state scholarships unconstitutional.[98] The courts ordered states to accept Black students in their state-supported White universities or create separate Black graduate schools. Even under court order, many Southern states found ways to deny African Americans admission at the graduate level.

The tendency for greater integration in graduate programs has continued to the present day, even at Black colleges. Many graduate programs at Black colleges are quite diverse, while their undergraduate programs are overwhelmingly Black.[99] For example, the law school entering class at North Carolina Central University in 2010 was 40 percent White, while the undergraduate program was still nearly all Black.[100]

When Morehouse College decided to move forward with a medical school, opinions differed about how supportive the Atlanta community would be. According to James Story, associate professor of anatomy in the Medical Education Program, "there were some dissenters, but by and large the majority of the White population in Atlanta accepted the school."[101] Whites, according to the Atlanta University feasibility study, felt that the medical school would "provide a logical and desirable source of much-needed black physicians, produce a quality student acceptable at any other existing medical school, . . . and assist in the reduction of health care need[s] in the Atlanta community, Georgia, and the Southeast."[102] Members of the Black community agreed with these sentiments, but they also thought that the addition of a new medical school would "reduce the problems of psychological distance and sociological isolation often felt by Southern Blacks desirous of entering the medical field . . . [and] increase the number of capable Black students attending medical school but who might not go to an all-White school due to financial problems."[103] According to Story: "Blacks in Atlanta were quite [politically] powerful during the early years of the medical program and still are. The city had a Black mayor and the effects of Martin Luther King Jr. were still quite profound."[104] Moreover, the majority of Black politicians in Atlanta had gone to Morehouse or Clark College.[105]

Charles Hatcher, then chief executive officer (CEO) of Emory Medical

Center, remembers a lot of support from the beginning for the idea of the medical school at Morehouse. From his perspective, "everybody thought this is a good idea. Emory and the University of Georgia are not recruiting as many minority students as we would have thought they could or hoped they could. When the idea of having a minority medical school that was a part of the Atlanta University Center and Morehouse College surfaced, it was clear cut, and everyone could jump on the bandwagon. I don't remember anyone in the Atlanta community objecting to the idea."[106] According to Bernard Hallman, associate dean at Emory, one of the reasons his school supported the Morehouse medical program was that Emory was worried that Georgia State University, which was rapidly expanding and was close to Grady Memorial Hospital, might create a medical school and serve as competition for Emory in the state, as well as competition for the use of Grady Hospital as a training site for its students.[107]

Relationship with Emory University

The creation of Morehouse's medical school was based on strong interracial cooperation; since its founding, the institution has benefited from cross-racial leadership. During the early years, when the medical school was merely an idea, Arthur Richardson, the White dean of Emory University's School of Medicine, was greatly involved. At the time, Richardson was the longest-serving medical school dean in the country. He used his prestige and experience to support the medical school idea. Richardson spoke out publicly, noting that Emory had not been successful in recruiting the number of Black students it desired. He thought perhaps it could make a contribution by helping Morehouse's medical school come into being.[108] In Charles Hatcher's opinion: "The institution is very sensitive to its social obligations, [it is] a very liberal type of a university, and it felt like we were not doing well at having [just] two or three students a year in Atlanta, so we were caught in a hard place. Every time we would identify somebody that could qualify for the Emory Medical School and meet our standards and requirements, they also met [the standards of] Harvard or Johns Hopkins or someplace where they could get a large scholarship."[109]

Of course, one of the reasons that Emory was not successful in recruiting Black students was that they were looking for the ideal student. Emory pursued African Americans with a 4.0 grade point average from Morehouse College or Xavier University. Unfortunately for Emory, these students would usually choose to enroll at Harvard University, the University of Pennsylvania, or Columbia University. Because Emory did not have the reputation, prestige, and history of an Ivy League institution—or the scholarship money—it had a difficult time luring the top African American students.[110]

Although Emory said that it could not attract Black students, in fact it was not admitting Blacks in any great numbers.[111] Many predominantly White colleges and universities hold fast to the idea that they desire yet cannot attract racial and ethnic minorities. This is one way to publicly support integration while maintaining a fairly homogeneous institution.[112] If Emory had truly wanted to enroll more African American students in its medical school, the administration could have altered their admissions requirements and provided developmental support aimed at making up for educational inequities. This is precisely what Morehouse and other Black colleges did and continue to do.

Although it could be argued that the creation of a Black medical school in a post-*Brown* era gives credence to the antiquated notion that separate could be equal (with equal funding), the unwillingness of White universities like Emory to take up the burden of closing achievement gaps shows that Black colleges had a unique mission and were truly needed. This argument holds true even today, given the dismal production of Black MDs by predominantly White medical schools. The idea behind Morehouse School of Medicine was not to create a segregated institution, but rather to provide opportunities for African Americans as well as others—and to provide more health services to low-income communities, making doctors the economic centers of these communities.

Morehouse College Seeks Support

During this period, NIH's Bureau of Health Manpower was part of the U.S. Department of Health, Education, and Welfare (HEW). With the support of Kenneth Endicott (the Bureau's director) and Bill Bennett, the Morehouse feasibility study was funded at $98,858 in February 1973.[113] The study revealed that Morehouse College had the academic strength, the administrative leadership, and the fundraising capacity to develop a medical education program.[114] Morehouse College's ability to organize and implement a two-year basic medical science curriculum was based on the college's success in running a premedical education program and its demonstrated achievements in the area of fundraising. Roughly 7 percent of the Black physicians in the

United States at the time had received their undergraduate education at Morehouse.[115] And, as noted earlier, Morehouse College was a leader in fund-raising among the Black colleges.

In June 1973, with the help of an $800,000 grant from the Bureau of Health Manpower, the planning process for a medical program at Morehouse College began, under the leadership of chemistry professor Joseph N. Gayles and with the assistance of biology professor Thomas C. Norris and director of development Alice G. Greene.[116] Greene was careful to downplay the fact that she was Hugh Gloster's daughter. She wanted to be recognized for her own capabilities, and her father was afraid of being accused of nepotism. In fact, she was an accomplished fundraiser and played a significant role in developing the medical school.[117] Another physician who was important to its start was Calvin A. Brown. Brown was an alumnus of Morehouse College ('52) and a close friend and supporter of Gloster's. As vice-chairman of the Morehouse board, Brown was a strong advocate for the medical program. In fact, Brown's basement was often used by Gloster, Gayles, Norris, Greene, and others for brainstorming sessions about the medical school.[118]

HEW employee Bill Bennett became a kind of ex-officio member of the planning team. He took a personal interest in the medical school at Morehouse and devoted many, many hours to making sure the endeavor succeeded.[119] In fact, Bennett helped Morehouse secure the $800,000 contract that supported planning for the medical school. The contract that Morehouse applied for was tailor-made for the institution. It called for an undergraduate college in a metropolitan city to develop a medical school; moreover, the college had to have limited resources and provide care for underserved populations. According to Bennett: "Morehouse was really the only one that could have done it, and when you looked at the contract you could tell it was for Morehouse. Everyone knew it."[120] After creating an opportunity for Morehouse to secure this contract, Bennett helped the Morehouse planning committee design a national model for developing a medical school.[121]

To assist the planning team, in 1974 Morehouse formed a committee that was composed of alumni of the college who held positions in academic medicine in various schools around the country. Louis W. Sullivan, a prominent alumnus and professor of medicine and physiology at Boston University's School of Medicine, was asked to be a part of that committee.[122] According to Sullivan: "Like many of my fellow alumni, I had serious questions about the wisdom of Morehouse College starting a medical school. Colleges don't start medical schools. Universities start medical schools, and very rich universities. Some very rich universities have decided they want nothing to do with a medical school—Princeton, MIT, and other institutions of that caliber. So when Morehouse College decided that they wanted to explore starting a medical school, as an alumnus in medical education, I was very concerned."[123] Indeed, not being affiliated with a university, with its sprawling professional schools, is a unique aspect of the Morehouse School of Medicine story.[124]

Approaching Governors and Legislators for Support

Despite some alumni skepticism, planning committee member Joseph Gayles, who was well connected in Atlanta and throughout Georgia, pushed on with the effort to found the school. He brought a copy of a 1969 National Institutes of Health report, which detailed the need for additional primary care doctors nationwide, to then governor Jimmy Carter. Along with others from Morehouse, Gayles used the report to convince Carter that he and the state should support the medical school.[125] Governor Carter did not need much convincing, however; he had heard about the medical school idea through his close friend Benjamin E. Mays, the stalwart former president of Morehouse. Carter said, "It was during my four years [1971–1975] as governor that the question of a medical school at Morehouse came up in the state legislature and in the budget committees."[126] At that time, according to Carter, "Georgia was making the change from a hundred years of so-called separate but equal towards a much more enlightened acceptance of a [U.S.] Supreme Court ruling." Carter thought the medical school idea was good for Georgia's Black citizenry. But more than that, it would benefit the state as a whole by providing quality medical care in low-income and rural areas. He used money from his Governor's Emergency Fund to help seed the new medical school. In his words: "My emergency fund was $2 million a year, which was quite a lot of money then; there were no restraints on how I spent the money. I could give a local city money to build a basketball gymnasium or a livestock barn or things of that kind. I often gave to interesting ideas, like the medical school, from that fund."

The timing was perfect for Morehouse in terms of approaching the local community and state government to support such a project. If it had waited much longer, Morehouse might have missed the opportunity, as Mercer University in Macon was also thinking about starting a medical school and looking for state support. According to Rhodes Haverty, "we got a lot of people from middle Georgia, and particularly around Macon—mainly Baptists; they were really pissed off with us because we wouldn't support them, we at the Medical Association, like we had supported Morehouse."[127] In Haverty's opinion, the people at Mercer thought, "We are a central part of Georgia, we're mostly White, we are good Southern Baptists—why did you support a Black school and not us?" He continued: "If both institutions had come to us at the same time, any one of the four possibilities could have happened. We could have turned them both down, we could have supported Mercer, we could have supported Morehouse, or we could have supported both of them. It's just that Morehouse came to us first, and the logic behind starting Morehouse was so compelling." Haverty, who is White, had access to state legislators that the Black administrators at Morehouse did not, and he used that access to assist the budding medical school.[128]

Haverty was convinced that the state needed physicians, but more acutely, it needed more Black physicians to take care of Georgia's Black population.[129] With his help, Morehouse was able to garner political support within the state and avoid any serious political problems. In his words, "I guess my own history with Morehouse is that I got organized medicine in Georgia to back the creation of a new medical school, and more importantly, a Black medical school."

Interestingly, Bill Bennett was also being pressured at the federal level by those who supported Mercer University's efforts to start a medical school. As he recalls:

> Senator Sam Nunn from Georgia called me to his office. Mercer had started to think about developing a medical school before Morehouse did, but by 1974, they could see that Morehouse was standing in the door and they were still working and planning. Senator Nunn told me, "From now on, when you go to Atlanta, you go to Morehouse in the morning and Mercer in the afternoon." He wanted me to spend equal time in the two schools. I said, "Sure, sure."[130]

Admittedly, Bennett was favoring Morehouse College. As an African American, Bennett said the project was close to his heart, and he felt he had a stake in the institution's success.

State Support Secured; Leadership Needed

After getting involved in the Morehouse College alumni committee in 1974, Louis W. Sullivan became "sold on the idea, the viability of this idea, the attractiveness of this idea, and the need for this institution, and the capability of the Atlanta University Center, with its six institutions, [in] forming an academic home for the medical school."[131] Sullivan's heartfelt connection to Morehouse helped turn him from doubter to believer. In his words: "With Morehouse, being an alumnus means you're part of the club. So I gave this idea some attention that I'm sure I would not have given it had it been from any other institution." After convincing himself that the idea had worth, Sullivan recommended a number of people whom he thought should lead the program, submitting a list of names to the planning committee. About three weeks later, Sullivan received a call from Joseph Gayles, who thanked him for submitting the names of 11 people who might head the medical program but said that "the list was not complete." According to Sullivan:

> Just as I was starting to respond, I was about to say, "What do you mean it's not complete!" I was angry. I had spent a lot of time developing this list. But then I realized what he was saying. I said, "Oh, no. I told you from the beginning I'm not a candidate. As an alumnus, I'm happy to consult and advise, but I'm very happy as a professor of medicine here at Boston University. I have three children, all born in Boston. They go up to New Hampshire in the winter to ski, and we go down to the Cape in the summer. I have a research laboratory and hematology fellows in training. So I'm not the person you want."

Upon hearing Sullivan's emphatic "No!" Gayles replied, according to Sullivan: "We thought you would have that response. The committee has instructed me to ask you—you're not a candidate, but would you be willing to come down to New York on September 14 to meet with the committee? We're going to have a series of meetings at the Hilton Hotel in New York. If you would come down and share your ideas with the committee about what you think such a school should look like, this would be very valuable." Sullivan responded: "All right, Joe. I'm willing to do this as long as it is very clear to you and the other members of the committee that I'm a consultant. I'm an alumnus. I'm not a candidate." Gayles replied, "Oh yes, we understand."

Sullivan attended the luncheon in New York, which was supposed to be finished around 2:30 p.m. However, when his wife, Ginger, who had driven with him from Boston for the day, called to pick him up, Sullivan asked her to come back in an hour. The meeting eventually came to a close at 4:00 p.m.[132] As Sullivan recounts, at the end, President Gloster of Morehouse, who was chairing the meeting, said:

> Dr. Sullivan, we know you are not a candidate, but I've been very impressed personally by our discussion today. I'm convinced in my mind that you're the man we

want. You're the man for this job. I can't speak for the committee, but I hope that as you drive back to Boston you will think about this. You would do your alma mater a great service, and the country a great favor, if you were to take this on.[133]

As Sullivan and his wife drove back to Boston, Ginger asked why her husband was silent. Sullivan replied, "Do you think you could consider the possibility of living in Atlanta?" She said: "I knew it! I knew it! I told you that they would want you there to set up the medical school."[134] Sullivan realized that he had "become totally seduced by the idea." Shortly afterward, he accepted the position, and he "hasn't regretted the decision for one moment."[135] According to Ginger, "we talked about it for a while, and I knew he liked a challenge and wanted to do it, so I agreed to move."[136]

James Story, the medical program's first faculty member, thought Sullivan was the "perfect guy" to lead the program. In his words:

> I had never heard such an eloquent speaker, and we needed a Dr. Sullivan type. He was the kind of guy who could talk with the governor, the mayor; he could get the state of Georgia to support the school, as well as the United States government to underwrite this new medical school. Lou was the consummate politician. He had credentials that Washington would respect.[137]

According to Ginger Sullivan, however, not everyone "was committed to having Lou as president of the medical school. The question was, 'Why do we need a Boston doctor to come down and organize the start of Morehouse School of Medicine? We have lots of doctors in Atlanta already.' "[138] Some very successful local doctors felt that they should have been chosen. However, the board thought that it took more than being a successful physician to start a medical school. Sullivan had been on many committees at the National Institutes of Health, had worked as a consultant to various medical schools, and was active in senior leadership at Boston University. He also had a national reputation for increasing the enrollment of minority students in medical schools in New England. For these reasons, the Morehouse board was convinced that he was the right person for the job.[139] Bill Bennett thought Sullivan was the perfect person to lead Morehouse School of Medicine because he had a big ego: "He came in to the New York meeting full of ego. I liked that. I saw a little bit of myself in him. He was a little cocky. I once told him, 'Lou, the reason I wanted you to be dean was because with your ego, like me, you'll die before you fail.' "[140]

CHAPTER THREE

Building His Bike as He Rides It

At a press conference on the day of Louis W. Sullivan's 1975 appointment to the position of dean of the Morehouse College Medical Education Program, President Hugh M. Gloster said, "We celebrate a tremendous triumph today, and we welcome you, Dr. Sullivan, for consenting to come and help make the Morehouse College Medical Education Program a reality."[1] Several prominent guests were at that press conference, including Arthur Richardson, the dean of Emory University, as well as Georgia's U.S. senators, Herman Talmadge and Sam Nunn.[2] Talmadge was a conservative senator, but he was not the ardent and vocal segregationist that his father had been. He was an astute politician, fully aware of the changing dynamics of the South and the influence of such figures as Martin Luther King Jr., U.S. Congressman Andrew Young, Joseph Lowery of the Southern Christian Leadership Conference, and others. Sam Nunn was a moderate to conservative Democratic senator from Georgia who tended to break with the party on social issues.[3]

According to Sullivan: "Talmadge and Nunn were supporting our school, which was quite profound. I, as a Black youngster growing up in Georgia, was quite familiar with Herman Talmadge's father, Eugene Talmadge, with his red suspenders and his political discourse of segregation."[4] Eugene Talmadge served three terms as governor of Georgia during the 1930s and 1940s. A staunch supporter of Jim Crow, he conducted a purge of the state's university system, removing a dean who he claimed was an integrationist and a Communist.[5] His son Herman started his career with a similar approach, opposing the *Brown v. Board of Education* decision and writing a pro-segregation book in 1955.[6] But Herman Talmadge's views evolved over time. The press conference was a sign of how much the South was changing, and of the interracial cooperation on which the medical school was built.[7]

Upon taking the position as dean, Sullivan said at the press conference: "I plan to do everything in my power to attract the best students, the best faculty, and to develop the best possible environment for teaching and learning. I am committed to finding new ways and models of training health professionals who can deliver quality medical care throughout the country."[8] Sullivan's ad-

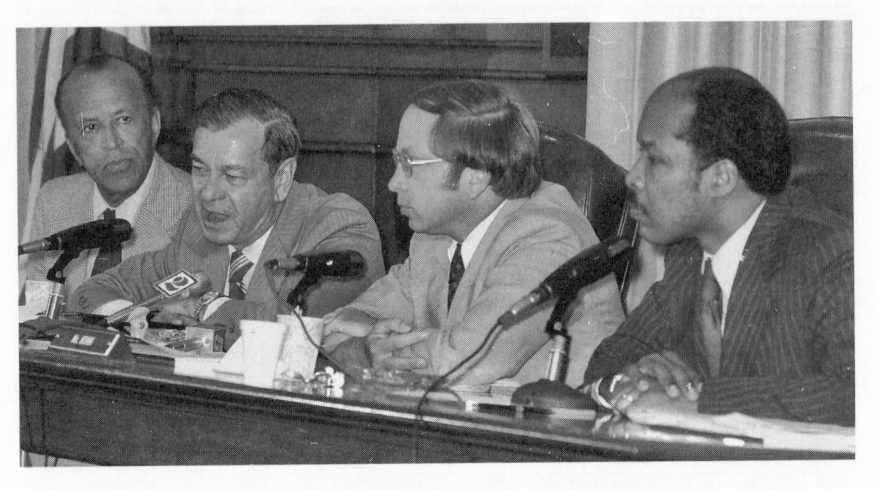

Press conference on Capitol Hill in Washington, D.C., November 1975. *Left to right,*
Hugh Gloster, U.S. Senators Herman Talmadge and Sam Nunn, and Louis W. Sullivan.

ministrative position was quite a change for a faculty researcher. No longer
was he responsible merely for his own professional success, but for the
growth and development of an entire group of physicians, students, and
teachers. In his words, "an administrator gets his or her gratification in the
long run in seeing the institution unfold and develop."[9] And Sullivan believed that his administrative role was all the more challenging, given the
stigma that had been placed on Black institutions in the past. "I wanted
to show the nation," he said, "that Black institutions could operate with the
same level of excellence as any other institution if given the resources. The
problem with so many Black institutions is that they have been starved for
resources."[10] Indeed, there is ample evidence that Black colleges received less
support from corporations and foundations as well as from the federal and
state governments.[11]

In Sullivan's view, the school had multiple missions. First, it had to produce excellent physicians—people who would be great scientists. Second, as
he noted above, it had to demonstrate that a Black institution could achieve
as much as any other institution if given the resources. Third, it had to respond to the feeling that African Americans have a responsibility to put their
shoulder to the wheel in order to make things happen. According to Sullivan:

> We as a nation have an unfortunate history of slavery, segregation, and discrimina-
> tion, and all of us have been victimized by that, Whites as well as Blacks. But let's
> get beyond that. Let's really show that every member of our society, whether you are

Black, White, Hispanic, every member can contribute positively to make this a better society if given the chance and if given the resources. So that's the larger story of Morehouse School of Medicine.[12]

Leadership Style: High Expectations

To accomplish all that he had by the age of 41, Louis Sullivan had maintained high expectations for himself. But what Sullivan had done so far, he had done as an individual faculty member, controlling his own schedule and research agenda. When the medical researcher took on the deanship of the Morehouse medical program, he also had high expectations for those he worked with and supervised. Gary MaGaha, who served under Sullivan as a special assistant and assistant professor of community health, said: "Lou is a penetrating leader. He is a perfectionist by nature. He is energized by challenges, and working for him is not something that anybody who is not totally committed to their lieutenant can do. If you don't have a lot of energy and you aren't there for him, you're in trouble." That said, MaGaha added: "I enjoyed working for him. It was my life. I slept with a legal pad by the side of my bed. My travel schedule was always his. Whatever he wanted me to do, I did those things in terms of assisting him, and it was challenging for me as a family man, but my family knew that I came here to assist with the building of the medical school."[13]

David Satcher, director of the Center for Primary Care at the medical school and former surgeon general of the United States, saw many leadership qualities in Sullivan: "Lou is the type of leader who inspired a lot of confidence in the people who worked under him. He was well connected politically. He used that as well as anybody I've seen to support the development of the school. Lou has this roaring voice. He has this great smile. And he meets with people directly and gains their respect and trust; people invest in you if they trust you."[14] Satcher also noted some characteristics that not everyone would find appealing: "He has a formal approach to him; not that he can't enjoy life, he's just formal. He has a strong ego. I know other people with big egos that I don't think as highly of as I do of Lou—but that's just who Lou is. He has a lot of self-confidence, and there's a real place for that when you're struggling to get something like this institution going." But all in all, Satcher felt, Sullivan's warmth and ardent belief in the Morehouse School of Medicine idea won people over: "He inspired confidence in the students, in the faculty, that they could be good. He had high standards from the beginning."

Part of Sullivan's strategy was to convince people that the medical school was a viable, important idea. As fundraiser Charles Stephens put it:

I had to meet him at the office every morning at 8 a.m. That's when we got started and set the schedule for the day, set the schedule for the week. And every day was a workday, Monday through Sunday. When others had days off, vacation days, Christmas Eve, that did not apply to us if something needed to be done. And if there was an instance where the medical school building was closed and there was no heating or air, we met at his house, in the kitchen, to get things done. It was a very uplifting experience.[15]

Perhaps Sullivan's work ethic is the reason prominent Atlanta doctor Asa Yancey Sr. referred to him as "the driving engine, the steam and everything else behind the success of Morehouse School of Medicine."[16] Gary MaGaha concurred: "I used to tell Lou that the brick and mortar of the school were held together with his blood. And that if we would cut him, he would probably bleed the school colors, not red."[17] As Angela Franklin, the former dean of students of the medical school, recalled: "It was a running joke that Lou was building his bike as he was riding it. To be able to create Morehouse School of Medicine from scratch is an amazing thing."[18] She added: "He was the kind of leader that would roll up his sleeves and get down with it and do whatever needed to happen. That's how he created something from nothing. He respected everyone's role and listened."[19]

Marjorie Smith, a beloved Morehouse School of Medicine faculty member who has been with the institution for years, said that Sullivan "wanted to be involved and take care of everything. When you have that kind of attitude, you want to make sure that you're on top of everything. And I think that was good because I don't know if anyone else would have taken ownership of the school; when you are starting a school, you need to take ownership."[20] The faculty who worked with Sullivan noted that he had a definite way of doing things, very high expectations of everyone, including himself, and he was not shy about letting people know so.[21]

Although Sullivan possessed the ability to "work a room" and had considerable charisma, he was not, according to board member Sarah Austin, "one of the boys." He wasn't the type to go out with the guys for a drink or to play golf. From Austin's perspective, Sullivan was single-minded in pursuit of his goals.[22] Sullivan basically agrees with this assessment of his personality and leadership, noting that the "school was a mission" to him and that he was focused on building it rather than socializing.[23]

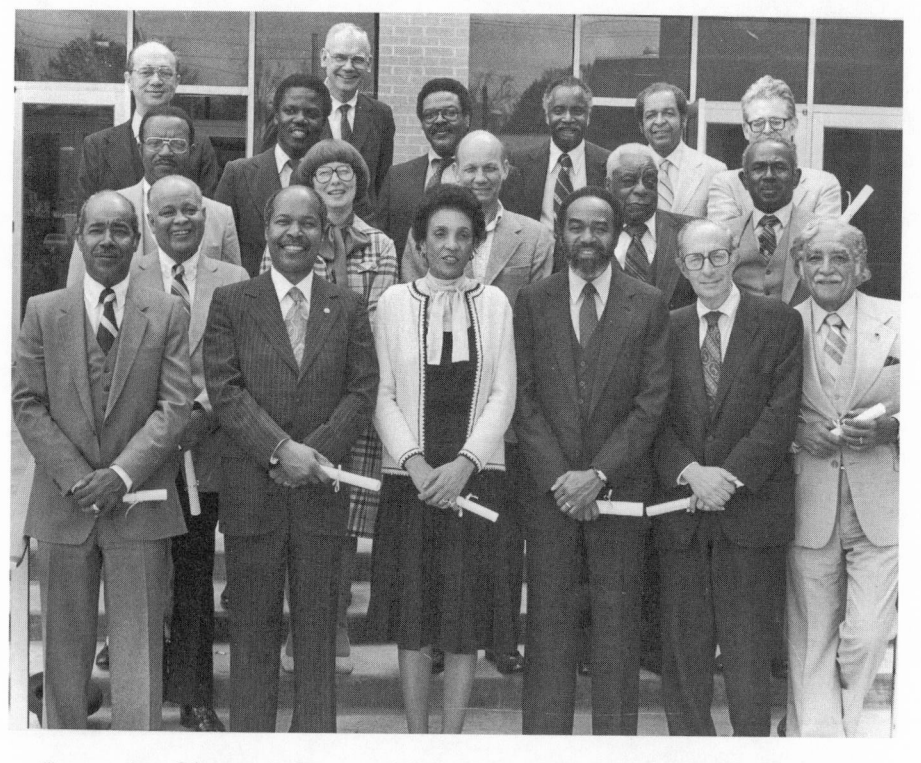

First meeting of the Board of Overseers for the Medical Education Program at Morehouse College, April 1976. *Left to right, bottom row*, Clinton Warner, Louis Sullivan, Sarah Austin (secretary of the board), Edgar Smith (chairman of the board), Morton Miller, Edward Mazique. *Second row*, Calvin A. Brown (vice-chairman, Board of Trustees, Morehouse College), Constance Menninger, Robert Forman, James B. Harris, Carleton Goodlett. *Third row*, James Palmer, Hugh Burroughs, Monroe Trout, Edward Saunders, Alphonso Overstreet, Clyde Phillips, and Pierre Galletti. Photograph courtesy of Roland Welmaker.

Despite his strong influence, the success of the medical program at Morehouse required the leadership of many people. According to Sullivan: "Leadership is not just one person. It's a group of people who provided different kinds of leadership that has made us the institution we are today."[24] Despite excellent leadership, there were also those within Morehouse College itself who initially had their reservations about the medical school, for several reasons. First, Black colleges typically don't have extensive resources.[25] Some questioned whether Morehouse College had the financial wherewithal to host a medical program. Second, there were those who wondered if the college had the administrative leadership structure to guide and staff the medical school. Lastly, some wondered if Morehouse had enough experience operating a large, complex institution.[26] Morehouse is a small, liberal arts college that has never enrolled more than 3,000 students and has roughly 150 faculty members. From Sullivan's perspective, "it's a good thing that I wasn't exposed to those questions before I took the job, because had I had time to think about that, I might still be trying to push vitamin B-12 across cell membranes in Boston rather than coming back to Atlanta to start a medical school."[27]

Humble Beginnings

Charles Stephens was an active member of the group championing the medical program and a fundraiser during the early years:

> It was amazing to be a part of a pioneering effort, and I think that all of the people who were involved in the school, faculty and others, felt this to be pioneering. That was the attitude. We had an interesting group of folks. I don't think I'd describe them as a motley crew, but a rather interesting group of young folks, people who were beginning their careers but also people who were well into their careers who were very, very respected in the field of medical education, people who had enormous achievement, people who had done work across the world. We had a staff that was fully integrated.[28]

One of Sullivan's goals for the medical school was to bring together faculty of all racial and ethnic backgrounds, as well as to have gender balance.

The program started in two brown trailers—with a total of 4,000 square feet—that sat between the Morehouse College science building and a classroom building. Various staff members were assigned to faculty recruitment, admissions, student affairs, and fundraising. When it came to recruiting faculty to staff the medical school, Sullivan looked for the best physicians and professors throughout the country, without regard to race. Early faculty members included Cyril Moore, chair of the Biochemistry Department; Jim Story, professor of anatomy; Bob Holland, chair of the Anatomy Department; Gordon Leitch, chair of the Physiology Department; and Gordon Bailey, professor of biochemistry. With support from the Rockefeller Foundation, Holland, Leitch, and Bailey had developed the Mahidol University School of Medicine in Thailand. The foundation helped recruit them to Morehouse and paid their full salaries during their first year there.[29]

One of Sullivan's concerns was how the interracial staff would get along. Would there be tensions and, ultimately, a separation into Black and White

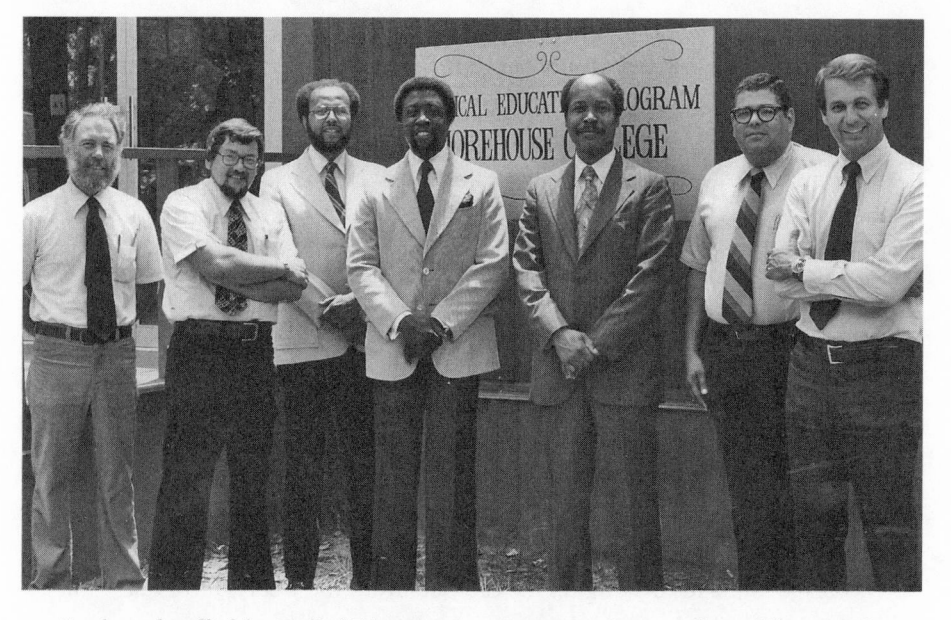

Faculty and staff of the Medical Education Program at Morehouse College, fall 1977. *Left to right*, Thomas Norris, Stephen Margolies, Joseph Gayles, James Storey, Louis Sullivan, Carter Marshall, and Gordon Bailey.

groups in the dining room, for example? He also wondered how the students, mostly Blacks, would react to the faculty, 50 percent of whom were White, owing to the shortage of minority medical faculty across the nation.[30] But there were never any major incidents among the faculty and students.

In the spring of 1976, the medical school recruited Beverly Allen, a librarian, from the Peoria campus of the University of Illinois College of Medicine. She was one of the first women on the all-male Morehouse campus, and her hiring posed some challenges for the new institution. As Louis Sullivan recalls: "We had to put in women's toilets for her and the female medical students. The only female toilet on the campus of Morehouse College was in the faculty lounge. And these were things which, frankly, us men never thought of at the time. But in retrospect, it's sort of obvious."[31]

A Limit on Space

Acquiring usable temporary space on the Morehouse College campus was difficult. For example, Allen called Sullivan one day and said, "When you get a chance, would you come over to my office? I want to show you something."

Sullivan made his way over to her office, which was part of the medical program's new library in the basement of Brawley Hall, one of Morehouse College's buildings. When he arrived, he commented on how nice the space was and asked Allen whether she liked it. "Oh, it is very nice," she said, "but why don't you just wait a minute." All of a sudden, there was a burst of loud music and noise. The Morehouse College band practiced right next to the medical program's library space. After weeks of negotiations, the Morehouse administration agreed to move the band practice.[32]

As the medical program's staff grew, space became a crucial issue, and in 1978 the new medical school acquired Sale Hall for its academic programs. Sale was the second oldest building on the Morehouse College campus and was renovated to house the anatomy laboratory, classrooms, faculty and staff offices, and a student lounge. The gross anatomy lab was in the basement. Such a lab required the use of cadavers for human dissection. David Mann— one of the early faculty members, along with Cyril Moore and Tom Norris— was responsible for picking up the cadavers from the Georgia mortuary and bringing them back to Morehouse in a truck.

The college mailroom was also in the basement of Sale Hall, and although the medical faculty members were used to cadavers, the postmistress, Miss Lamar, was not.[33] A fixture of the college since Sullivan was a student in the 1950s, this venerable lady was a feisty disciplinarian. She was known for keeping a watchful eye on students and would threaten to call their parents if she saw them doing something wrong, even though it was not officially her job.

One day in June 1978, when Sullivan arrived at work, Lamar was waiting to see him. She said, "Dr. Sullivan, is it true? Is it true that there are going to be dead people down the hall from me?" Sullivan responded, "Well, Miss Lamar, we are going to have our gross anatomy laboratory down there, but you won't know anything about it." Miss Lamar blurted out, "Dead people?!" Sullivan said, "Well, I wouldn't call them that." He was trying to find a way to sugarcoat the situation, but he was failing miserably. Miss Lamar said, "Dr. Sullivan, I can't have that. I can't have dead bodies down here by the mailroom." Sullivan responded, "Miss Lamar, you won't smell anything or see anything." But Miss Lamar was not going to stand for having to work next to dead bodies. She said, "Oh no, I can't have that!" and went straight to President Gloster's office.[34]

Sullivan phoned ahead to alert Gloster that Miss Lamar was on her way. Gloster said he would take care of her, calm her down and explain the situa-

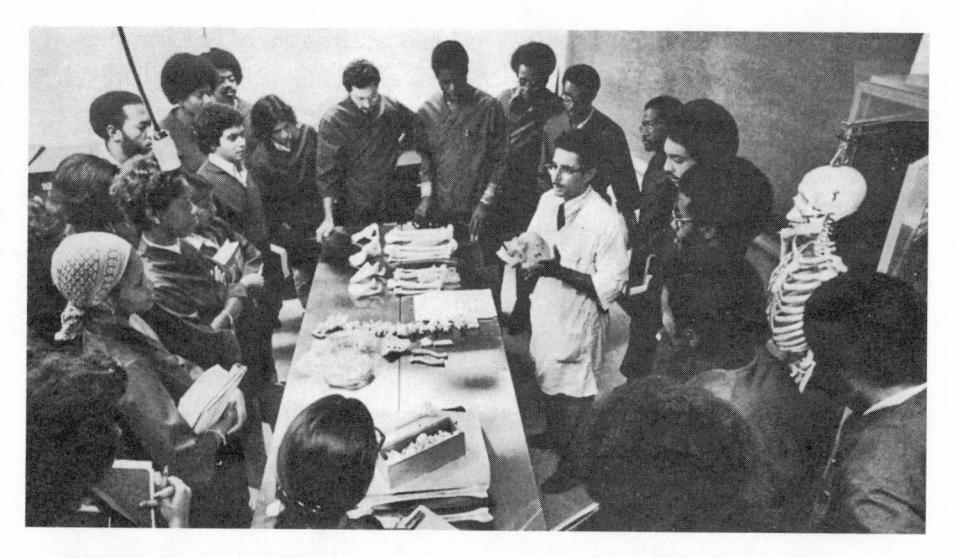

Professor Raymond Hayes on the first day of Gross Anatomy Laboratory, September 1978.

tion. He gave her his assurances that he would "take care of things." But nothing happened. Then, in August 1978, 10 days before the start of gross anatomy instruction, as Sullivan recalled: "We wheeled in the cadavers. They were on gurneys covered by white sheets. And the moment we wheeled those bodies in, Miss Lamar left the building, never to return." In fact, Miss Lamar successfully petitioned to move the student mailboxes to another Morehouse building.[35] Starting a medical school at a small college with deep traditions and long-tenured staff proved challenging, to say the least.

Space was also short in supply for the program's library and administrative offices. The basement of Brawley Hall housed the medical school's library and multimedia center, which was directed by Beverly Allen. The school's administrative offices were first located in the trailers, and then in Atlanta University's Harkness Hall, which also housed the Morehouse College administration.[36] According to former Board of Trustees member Delutha King: "In the early years, recruiting staff and faculty was a continuing challenge, and making provisions for the students in those early days was also very difficult. We didn't have the space for them."[37] By the summer of 1979, the medical college was bursting at the seams, and the institution renovated a nearby apartment building to accommodate faculty offices and student classrooms.[38] Mann recalled working in the building, a block away from Sale Hall: "The apartments were unbelievable. They were rodent infested, and there was a huge rat that used to come out in front of the apartment complex. He used to come out of the storm sewer, and he'd graze there on the grass. Seriously, he was as big as a small dog. He'd graze there, day in, day out." In Mann's opinion, "you had to have a certain personality to tolerate, to survive in this environment during the early days; things kept getting better and better, but you had to be patient."[39]

Mann recalled an incident involving the Laboratory Building—or the "tin building" as some early faculty and staff members affectionately called the prefabricated metal structure. It was built to house research and teaching laboratories for the medical school, using aluminum siding to minimize its cost. Mann was the radiation safety officer and was responsible for the storage of radioisotope waste from the laboratories. One evening, quite late at night, he received a call telling him that someone had driven a car into the "tin building" at high speed, plowing straight into the radioisotope storage area. "The firemen wouldn't go into the building because they were afraid it was unsafe," Mann said, "so I had to drive down and assure them that the level of isotopes that we had in there was relatively low. Things were a little loose in those days, some 25 years ago."[40]

The medical program had the "tin building" erected on Morehouse College land in order to house research labs. Although the main mission of the medical school was primary care, there was a growing interest among faculty members in conducting basic biomedical research.[41] To finance the research building, Morehouse College asked the assistance of a local bank, which in essence owned the structure. For five years the College leased the building from the bank at a steep rate—roughly $200,000 a year. At the end of the five years, the bank sold the building to Morehouse for one dollar. Basically, the college paid for the building through the lease. The unorthodox nature of this arrangement came to Louis Sullivan's attention when he was visiting with one of Georgia's state senators, Al Holloway. A White legislator from Albany, Georgia, Holloway was reviewing the medical school's budget when he asked: "What is this lease of space you have here? Two hundred thousand dollars; what kind of building is that?" Sullivan responded, "Well, that's the building for laboratory research." Holloway replied, "Damn, that's a lot." At that point, Sullivan realized he had to come clean about the arrangement with the bank. He said, "Well, Senator Holloway, the reality is that the bank put up this building and we are leasing it in order . . . " Holloway interrupted him: "Stop right there. Don't tell me anything more. I don't want to hear this." The senator realized that he had uncovered a scheme developed by Morehouse

College and the bank, since the small, Black college did not have enough money to pay for the building outright. To avoid being tied to any wrong-doing, or being forced to investigate the transaction, Senator Holloway, a friend of Morehouse College, chose to simply ignore what he heard.[42]

Moving Forward, Raising Money

To avoid the kind of financial jeopardy exemplified by the "lease" on the lab building, the Morehouse board knew it had to make some changes. The first priorities were the organization's identity and its fundraising strategy. In the fall of 1977, the Board of Overseers of the Medical Education Program and the Board of Trustees at Morehouse College voted to rename the program the School of Medicine at Morehouse College. James Schofield, the secretary of the Liaison Committee on Medical Education (LCME), recommended this change. To represent the institution, they developed a new logo, which included both traditional symbols of medicine and symbols of Atlanta. The central form in the logo, a flame, represented "the light of knowledge," and in that flame was the letter *A*, representing Atlanta. The wings surrounding the flame symbolized a phoenix rising from the ashes—a reference to the fact that Atlanta was burned to the ground during the Civil War and rose up again. The form in the middle of the circle represents the tree of life and is entwined with a serpent, which is the traditional symbol of medicine as a healing art. The words at the base of the symbol detail the institution's goals: "The achievement of excellence; knowledge of medicine; service to those who need medical care; and wisdom of man and his environment."[43] Equipped with a representative logo and a mission dedicated to primary care and service in urban and rural areas, the new medical program set out to raise money to lay the groundwork for recruiting its first class.

Through the 1970s there was a continued shortage of physicians in the South, especially in areas with large concentrations of minorities. According to a report by the U.S. Department of Health, Education, and Welfare, in 1977 the number of physicians per capita in all the states in the Southeast except Florida was below the national average.[44] There was a particularly acute shortage of primary care physicians in rural and inner city areas. More-over, the number of African Americans and other minority students entering medical school declined from 7.2 percent to 6.8 percent between 1975 and 1977.[45] The mission of the medical school, which called for it to counter these trends, included the following: train medical students as primary care doc-

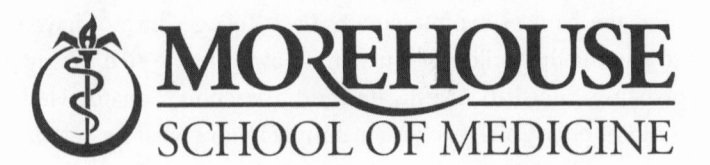

The 1981 logo for the Morehouse School of Medicine.

tors to work in underserved rural areas and the inner city; hire a faculty that is committed to teaching and research; incorporate in the curriculum those elements of the humanities and social sciences that will increase student understanding of, and appreciation for, the influence of personal and social problems that accompany patient reactions to illness; educate students who are academically talented and also those who require academic support; and recruit students from rural, inner city, and socially and economically disadvantaged backgrounds.[46]

As Morehouse School of Medicine was coming into its own, it had to contend with the same issue as many other medical schools—that of balancing its teaching and research missions. Medical schools seek to produce practitioners but, at the same time, medical school faculty members seek to be on the cutting edge of discovery and bring in research dollars. In the words of historian Larry Cuban, "the dominant belief that professors can play starring roles both in the classroom and in a scholarly discipline has become a surrogate battlefield for reconciling the inherent dilemmas within the university-college hybrid and the mixed purposes of the professional school."[47] The leadership of the Atlanta-based medical school made a conscious choice to put teaching and clinical practice first, but they also emphasized basic and clinical-oriented research.

In order to achieve its goals and secure accreditation from the Liaison Committee on Medical Education, the chief accrediting organization for medical schools, the school was required to raise $10 million. Compared to fundraising goals for other medical schools in the United States, this does not seem like a large sum, even at the time.[48] However, according to Charles Stephens, the institution's first fundraising officer, Morehouse's board was not fully developed: "There were some people on the board who were very capable, but it was new and they were new. So we didn't have a board that was used to working together for a long time."[49] He also observed that the institution's funders included the state and federal governments, corporations, and foundations, but no wealthy individuals. According to Stephens: "Corpora-

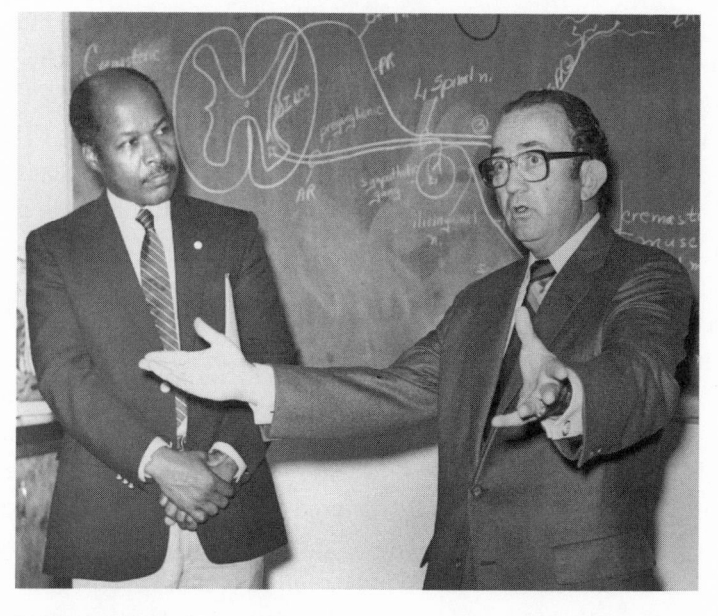

Louis W. Sullivan (*left*), with James Sammons, MD (*right*), executive director of the American Medical Association during Sammons's visit to the School of Medicine at Morehouse College, October 1977, to express the support of the AMA for the development of the Morehouse School of Medicine.

tions were hesitant. It was an undergraduate school trying to put a medical school in place, a two-year medical school, in an environment where most of the intelligence about medical schools in 1977 said we don't need another one."[50] Out of all the medical schools in the United States, none were affiliated with a small college; they either stood alone or were part of a larger university.[51]

Eventually, the medical program had to secure money from the state. This was tricky, according to Stephens: "How do you get state money for a private institution?" He then explained their strategy:

> The arrangement was that the grant would be made to the Board of Regents of the University of Georgia, and the money would then pass to the Southern Regional Education Board (SREB). There was a purchasing agreement for the SREB to support the development of a school of medicine in Georgia to increase the number of physicians in the state. So the money went from the state to the Board of Regents of Georgia to the SREB to Morehouse College. One million dollars annually for five years, and the accreditation was approved and things were rolling.[52]

Research grants from the National Institutes of Health (NIH) and other federal agencies are a significant source of support for all medical schools. According to sociologists Christopher Jencks and David Riesman, "the fact that
most congressmen have a relative who died of cancer . . . makes NIH relatively affluent."[53] In their book, *The Academic Revolution*, the sociologists suggest that the NIH leadership uses its influence to channel money to medical
schools in particular. However, to be eligible to receive federal support, a
medical school must be accredited by the U.S. official accrediting agency for
medical education, the Liaison Committee on Medical Education (LCME).
Beginning in 1973, the LCME required that all existing two-year medical
schools (Dartmouth College; University of Nevada, Las Vegas; University of
North Dakota; University of South Dakota) and any new two-year medical
schools had to have a plan, with timetables, to develop into an MD degree–
granting program. The LCME also required that two-year medical programs
have legal contracts with MD degree–granting institutions to guarantee that
their graduates would be accepted into the third year of medical school after
successfully completing the two-year curriculum. These requirements
spurred Morehouse School of Medicine to develop an MD degree–granting
program as soon as possible.[54]

Gaining provisional accreditation was one of the critical events in the
school's history, Sullivan said: "It meant we were really in business, and
we could admit our first class." The school received that standing from the
LCME in the spring of 1978, which helped in its efforts to organize and develop a two-year medical school, with transfer agreements with four-year
medical schools.[55] The school would not be eligible for full accreditation until
it began to offer a four-year medical program in 1985.

Getting the provisional accreditation in the spring complicated the process of recruiting the first class. All medical schools send out letters of acceptance to applicants by January 1 each year, but in 1978, Morehouse was
not able to send out its letters until April, after receiving the provisional accreditation. Thus the incoming charter class was made up of students who
had not been accepted by other medical schools.[56]

Throughout its history, Morehouse's medical school has admitted some
students who might not have been accepted at more elite schools, because
the administration believed that ratcheting up admissions requirements in
an attempt to compete with other medical schools would counteract its mission of recruiting students of color. For example, two of the Morehouse
School of Medicine's most prominent alumni were not admitted to any med-

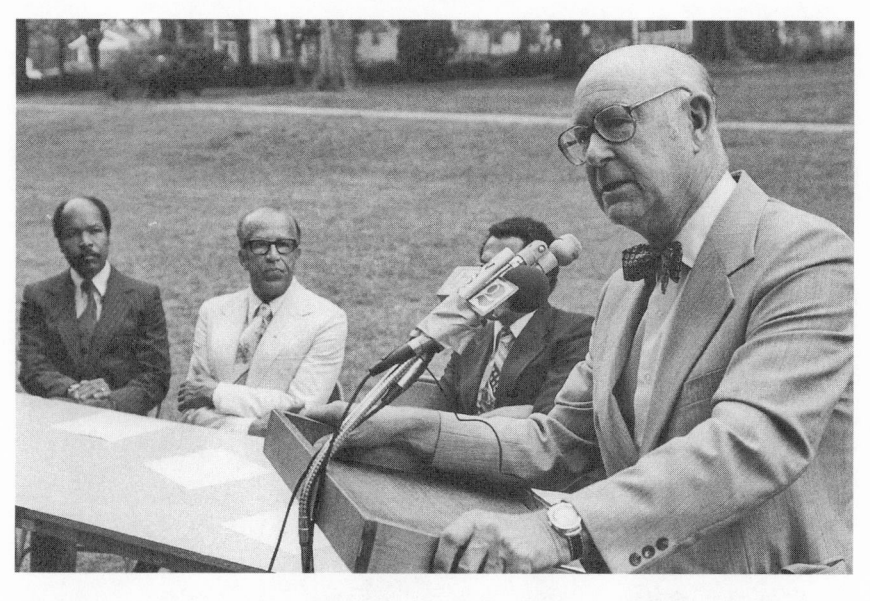

Press conference announcing the receipt of provisional accreditation of the School of Medicine at Morehouse College by the Liaison Committee on Medical Education, April 1978. *Left to right*, Dean Louis Sullivan, President Hugh Gloster, James Carter of the Medical College of Georgia, and Dean Arthur Richardson of Emory University.

ical schools the first time they applied. One is Regina Benjamin, a MacArthur "Genius" Award recipient and U.S. Surgeon General under President Barack Obama; the other is Wayne Riley, the president of Meharry Medical College. According to Sullivan, "the medical school offers students opportunities; we've always been flexible going in, in terms of admissions, but rigid going out, in terms of our graduation standards."[57]

In the spring of 1977, the Georgia General Assembly appropriated another $1 million to aid the medical school. Governor George Busbee and Lt. Governor Zell Miller, who made education a hallmark of their leadership, shepherded the appropriation, and, happily, the Senate and House appropriations committees supported it.[58] To celebrate the appropriation, U.S. Senators Talmadge and Nunn hosted a luncheon to introduce the medical school to the business and civic leaders of Atlanta and Georgia.[59]

Even this significant state support, however, didn't fill the medical program's needs. So in 1977, Louis Sullivan, along with "Daddy" King (Martin Luther King Sr.) and Morehouse College President Emeritus Benjamin E. Mays, went to Washington, D.C., to meet with then president and fellow Georgian Jimmy Carter.[60] They asked Carter to provide an annual federal ap-

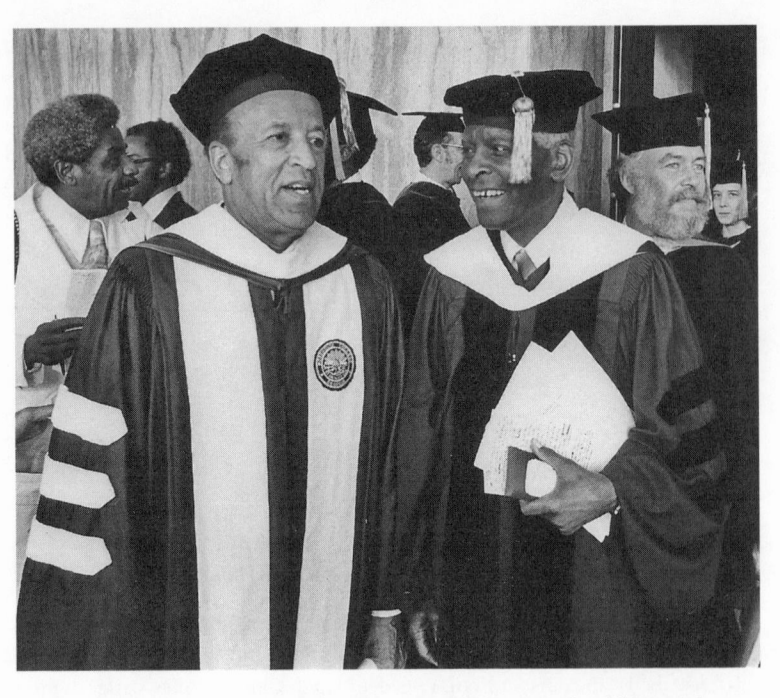

Morehouse College President Hugh M. Gloster (*left*) is congratulated by President Emeritus Benjamin E. Mays (*right*) after the inaugural convocation of the School of Medicine at Morehouse College, September 1978. Photograph courtesy of Bud Smith.

propriation for Morehouse School of Medicine similar to the federal support given to Howard and Gallaudet universities—institutions that had historically received a special appropriation because of the unique populations they served—African Americans and deaf people, respectively.[61] The three influential African American leaders made the case to Carter that Morehouse was a minority school and, as such, provided a great service to the nation by producing a significant number of African American doctors. President Carter asked his budget director, Burt Lance, to work on the issue.[62] Unfortunately, certain key members of Congress were not sympathetic to this type of appropriation; they felt that the annual federal support for Howard and Gallaudet had been a mistake and "were not about to establish another agreement of this nature."[63] Howard University's original charter was enacted by Congress in 1867 and signed into law by President Andrew Johnson. The charter designated Howard as "a University for the education of youth in the liberal arts and sciences." In 1879, Congress approved a special appropriation to the institution, and in 1928, the university charter was amended to include an an-

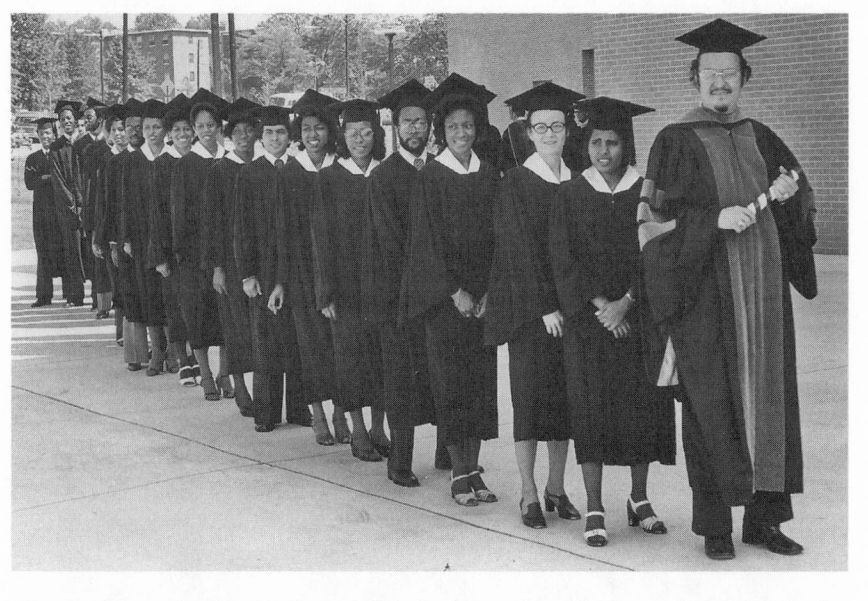

Charter class processional to the Martin Luther King Chapel for the convocation, School of Medicine at Morehouse College, September 1978. Photograph courtesy of Bud Smith.

nual federal appropriation.[64] Similarly, Congress issued and President Abraham Lincoln authorized a charter in 1864 to Gallaudet University, and since then the institution has received an annual appropriation equaling 70 percent of its operating budget.[65]

In President Carter, the Morehouse leaders found a sympathetic ear. The Georgia native had dedicated a substantial amount of his time as president to health care issues. His plans for health care reform were ambitious and included expanding health insurance coverage and reducing hospital costs. With the help of Senator Edward Kennedy, he nearly succeeded in passing a hospital cost–containment bill; the legislation passed the Senate but ran aground in the House after a huge lobbying effort by the hospital industry. Not until 2010, under President Barack Obama, would the United States see comprehensive health care reform.[66]

The Morehouse leaders offered a more modest but very effective way to expand health care coverage—by training physicians to serve the populations with the greatest need. Although Carter was not able to secure an arrangement similar to Howard's and Gallaudet's, he had Burt Lance investigate other options. Lance was particularly enthusiastic in his support of the School of Medicine at Morehouse College, as he, too, hailed from Georgia. Accord-

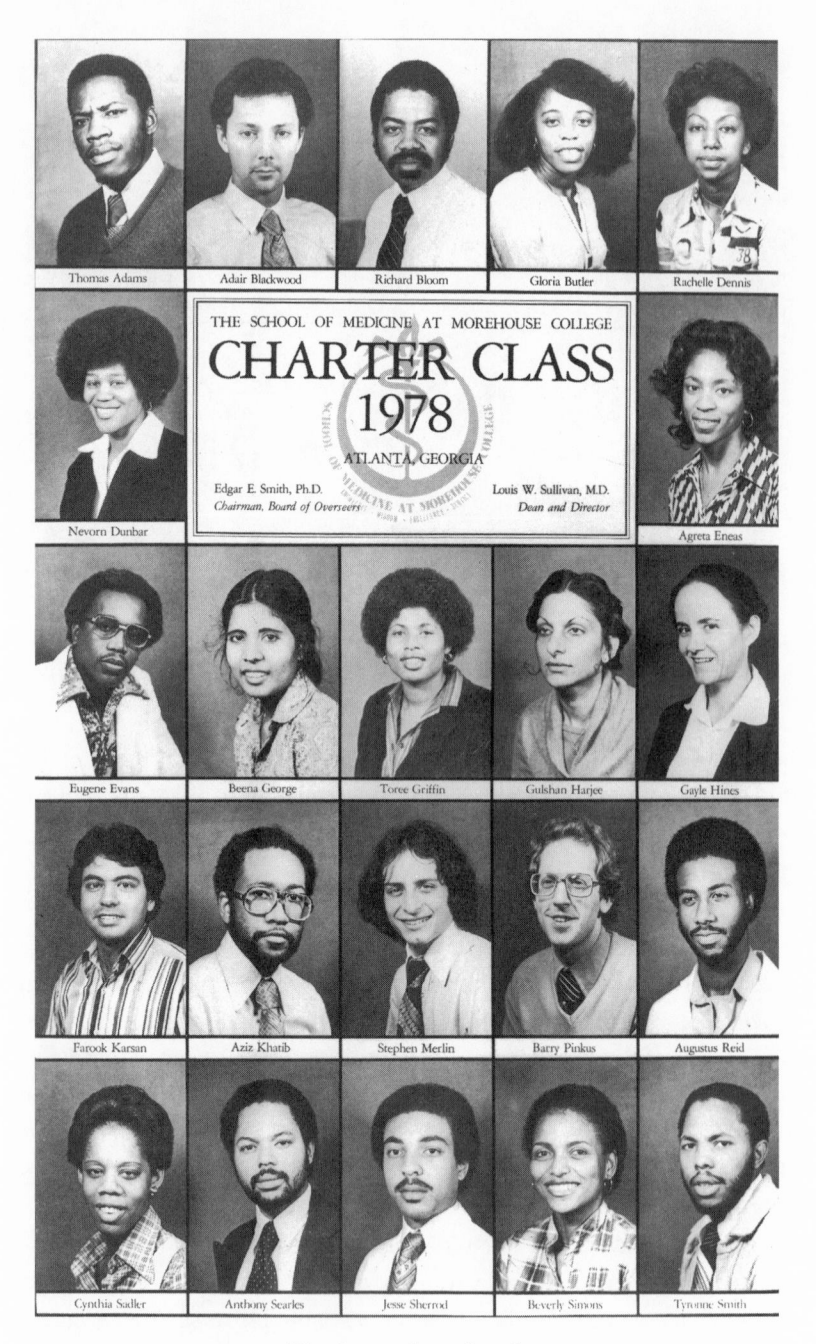

The charter class of 1978.

ing to Carter: "He was very familiar with Morehouse, and he saw Morehouse as a symbol of progress within the African American community. It was a symbol of higher education, and the excellence of their academic standards was very high."[67] In addition, Lance had been the chairman of the board of Calhoun National Bank in Atlanta before he became Carter's budget director, and he was very well acquainted with the Atlanta fundraising landscape.[68] According to Sullivan, "Burt Lance was quite supportive, and the medical school received several federal grants during President Carter's administration despite not being able to secure a regular federal appropriation like that of Howard and Gallaudet."[69]

Also instrumental in helping to garner federal money for Morehouse was U.S. Representative Andrew Young, who later served as ambassador to the United Nations and mayor of Atlanta. As a congressman (1973–1977), he was briefed on Morehouse College's plans to develop the medical school and was "really excited about it." In Young's words: "I jumped at the opportunity to work with Lou Sullivan and helped set up a meeting with him, Ted Kennedy, and Herman Talmadge. They agreed to add a $10 million appropriation to a particular bill to support the school. Interestingly, the bill did not mention Morehouse by name."[70] This situation was very much like the early planning contract that Bill Bennett designed for Morehouse. Andrew Young went on to say:

> It would have been difficult to put $10 million in the bill for one college. Basically the line in the bill said, "Ten million dollars to begin a medical school that sought to serve citizens in areas that were underserved in inner cities and small towns of America." It was really general, but at the same time it could have only applied to Morehouse, and so the money went directly to Morehouse.[71]

Of note, the coming together of conservatives and liberals in support of Morehouse School of Medicine was, and continues to be, one of the institution's strengths.

Charles Stephens recalled the difficulties that Sullivan faced during the early years, both in trying to raise funds and in trying to convince people that another medical school was needed.[72] For example, Stephens remembered a luncheon that Sullivan attended in New York, hosted by Monroe Trout, the medical director of Sterling Drug Company. It was a gathering of medical directors of major drug corporations throughout the city. Sullivan was making a presentation about the medical program to the group when "a young guy from one of the drug companies interrupted him to speak. He quoted from a report by Clark Kerr, which affirmed that there was not a need for another medical school."[73] Sullivan stopped, referenced the report, referenced the page on which this conclusion had been reached, and referred the young fellow to another chapter that pointed to a significant need for medical personnel in small communities, rural communities, and minority communities. He then resumed his speech as if nothing had happened.[74] Clearly, Sullivan was up to the task of defending Morehouse. He remained cool and effective under questioning, explaining in nuanced fashion how it was possible to support this medical school while acknowledging the glut of medical institutions overall.

One reason Sullivan was so well versed in the specifics of Kerr's report is that he had met with its author immediately after its release. Written by Carnegie-sponsored researcher Clark Kerr, who was also the president of the University of California system, the report initially did not support the development of a Black medical college. Recognizing that this was a problem, Hugh Gloster, who knew Kerr, sent Sullivan to California to meet with him. Sullivan discussed the implications of the report for Black colleges and Black doctors; he said there might be a glut of White doctors, but there was still a shortage of Black doctors, especially primary care physicians and those interested in working in inner city and rural areas. Kerr acknowledged "not having the right information."[75] After the conversation with Sullivan, Kerr issued a correction to the report, noting that Morehouse School of Medicine and the other Black medical schools were doing an important service by producing Black doctors, who were greatly needed across the country.

Kerr's retraction is significant, especially since the report was sponsored by the Carnegie Foundation—a funder that had a mixed reputation among Black college leaders. The foundation had given significant support to Black colleges over time, but it had also sponsored a damaging study conducted by Christopher Jencks and David Riesman in 1967 that labeled most Black institutions as "academic disaster areas."[76] The repercussions of this study sent Black colleges into a tailspin, with negative publicity in national news venues and questions raised everywhere about the viability of Black colleges overall. Soon, however, Black college leaders organized themselves to rebut the study's conclusions. Morehouse's President Gloster was a leader among those refuting Jencks and Riesman's claims, writing several nationally published op-eds, including one for *Time* magazine. Clearly, Black college leadership, and Gloster in particular, had become savvy about the influence of foundation-sponsored research in the field of higher education.[77]

In dealing with the Kerr report, President Gloster's connections proved very helpful to Sullivan. In fact, Gloster used his influence a great deal during the medical school's early years, accompanying Sullivan on fundraising trips and introducing him to big names in Atlanta. "He knew the folks who ran Atlanta and Georgia," said Gloster's wife, Yvonne.[78] Thanks to Gloster's relationships with the editorial staff of the *Atlanta Constitution*, the small college was able to keep the cause of the medical school in front of the general public; such publicity helped it garner widespread support and funds.[79]

Despite his self-confidence, Sullivan was a rookie when it came to fundraising. He hadn't done it as a professor, and he wasn't used to the sting of rejection. In July 1975, Gloster took Sullivan to see Boisfeuillet Jones, the head of the Coca-Cola–funded Woodruff Foundation, to ask him to support the medical school. Jones was cordial, but at the very start of the meeting he said: "Well, Dr. Gloster, I need to tell you and Dr. Sullivan that I wish you well with this medical school, but we are heavily in support of Emory Medical School. We don't have the resources to support more than one medical school. So you can't count on us as a source of support."[80] According to Sullivan: "Boy, that was a real downer. I was just starting to learn about fundraising, which, at that time, I didn't like."[81] He continued:

> It was my introduction to the eight-hundred-pound gorilla here in Atlanta—if you don't have the support of Woodruff in Atlanta, not only are you lacking those dollars, since they are the largest foundation, but it raises a question in the minds of other people. They say, "Gosh, if Woodruff is not supporting this, then maybe this is not as solid as we thought."

Fortunately, a year later, Sullivan was able to convince the Woodruff Foundation to provide funds for the medical program. Morehouse received a $250,000 grant to help purchase the institution's first two acres of property for its campus. During the grant period, Sullivan spent considerable time telling the Morehouse medical school story to the program officers at Woodruff and letting them know that their money was well spent. Over the course of the school's history, it has received many grants from the Woodruff Foundation, in spite of the fact that Emory is the foundation's primary beneficiary.[82] According to Clinton Warner, former board chair of Morehouse School of Medicine: "Lou was an excellent fundraiser and an excellent representative of the school. Wherever he went, he represented it well."[83] By 1978 Sullivan had raised $15 million, including $2.1 million from the federal government and $5 million from the state of Georgia.[84]

The Josiah Macy Jr. Foundation in New York was also generous to the medical school over the years, in terms of money as well as a willingness to make introductions. John Bowers, who was president of the Foundation in the 1970s and 1980s, was helpful to Sullivan during his early years at Morehouse. Bowers hosted a luncheon in New York in the fall of 1975 to introduce Sullivan to the foundation community in that city—including organizations such as the Rockefeller and Ford foundations, which had a long and complex history of supporting Black higher education.[85] According to Sullivan, "there were 30 to 40 people at the luncheon, and the purpose was to introduce all of them to the new medical school that was developing in Atlanta."[86] Bowers told the foundation leaders about the national shortage of Black physicians and noted that the Morehouse medical program focused on minority medical education. He made it clear that Sullivan would be following up with each of the luncheon participants afterward. Bowers also made introductions for Sullivan at the Pew Foundation in Philadelphia and the Kellogg Foundation in Battle Creek, Michigan. According to Sullivan, as well as the historical record, the Macy Foundation has been a fundamental supporter of the school; although its grants were small ($25,000–$250,000), this foundation sponsored conferences and publications for the medical school that helped offset its costs and bring it publicity. The Macy Foundation's support was also crucial because it was a recognized leader in the medical education world and paved the way for others to help fund the new medical school.

In April 1976 the medical school also established a Board of Overseers. This board consisted of a network of state and national supporters and potential donors who believed in the Morehouse School of Medicine idea. To chair the board, Morehouse chose Edgar Smith, professor of biochemistry at the University of Massachusetts School of Medicine. Smith was very familiar with the inner workings of both medical schools and Black colleges, having attended historically Black Tougaloo College for his undergraduate degree. Along with Sullivan, he recruited doctors, businessmen, and philanthropists from around the nation and from both the Black and White communities to serve on the board and bring attention to the institution.

To raise money and promote the institution, Sullivan and his wife, Ginger, would host small dinner parties at their home, inviting the trustees to join them. According to Andrew Young, this became a widespread practice among Black leaders because of segregation: "We couldn't host dinners in hotels or in fine restaurants during the era of segregation and for years after it. So everything was done in the home. Even though restaurants were integrating, there was something special about meeting in someone's home."[87] The gatherings at the Sullivans' home were always integrated, Young said, adding: "The people who are most successful, in their time in this town, have integrated parties and gatherings. People who are successful don't segregate in their social lives or in their business lives." This was "a strength of Lou Sullivan's—he reached across racial lines to work with folks."[88]

Ginger Sullivan was also instrumental in founding a giving circle, called the Friends of Morehouse School of Medicine, that helped to raise money for student scholarships. The Friends group, whose members were wives of business and political leaders in Atlanta, would host an annual dinner in one of Atlanta's finest hotels and sell sponsorships and tables to supporters. They would honor high-profile individuals, such as legislators, society women, and business leaders. The group also sent out letters soliciting funds. They were an enthusiastic and effective group, and they raised nearly $500,000 for scholarships over 10 years.[89]

Another creative method of raising money was through capitation funds— a per capita allocation for each Georgia resident enrolled at the institution per year, which Morehouse School of Medicine received because of the nationwide shortage of physicians. The federal government offered such funds especially to medical schools that were willing to expand their class size and accommodate the need for more physicians. Additional funds were available to schools that enrolled out-of-state students coming from states that lacked the capacity to provide their medical education. For example, during its early years, Morehouse School of Medicine received capitation support from the states of Alabama and New York for residents enrolled at the institution. These students would complete two years of their medical education at Morehouse and then transfer to a school in their home state. Capitation funds were quite helpful to the overall budget, because the medical school not only received the money, but the students paid full tuition. Morehouse School of Medicine also attempted to set up capitation agreements with New Jersey and California, but these states preferred to keep their students and tuition dollars at home. As the shortage of doctors came to an end, the capitation programs were discontinued.[90]

A First Class of Students

In September 1978, the School of Medicine at Morehouse College officially began operation as a two-year program in the basic medical sciences, admitting its first class of 24 students and boasting as its primary mission "the training of physicians who will establish practices for the medically under-served minority and socioeconomically disadvantaged in rural America and the inner cities."[91] James Story, an early faculty member, recruited the pro-gram's first class.[92] His recollections are as follows:

> I wanted our first class—our first students—to know that they shared the burden of getting this school off the ground. You know, the first African American medical school started in the twentieth century. I wanted them to feel that history. I tried to instill in them the desire to excel, not just to make it but to excel, because that was the legacy of Morehouse College as laid down back in the days of Dr. Benjamin Mays.[93]

To fill the first class, Story was looking for students who were "aggressive academically" and those who would "fit the environment and who wanted to be trailblazers, not in the sense of trying to say, 'I'm the first who did this,' but who could go through the rigors of being the first. That's not easy to do." The students also had to have "a thick skin, and they had to really want to do something for their race and for their nation, because that's why the medical school was founded." As many of the early supporters and administrators for the medical program were Morehouse College graduates, they were commit-ted to preserving the Morehouse brand and, in fact, improving on it with the addition of a professional school. The first class at the medical school was integrated: 14 out of 24 students were Black, 6 were White, and 4 were South Asian. Moreover, 14 students were male and 10 were female. From the begin-ning, there was always a commitment to bringing in a class that boasted gender, racial, and ethnic diversity.[94]

Turmoil amid Success

Although the recruiting of the first class of students in 1978 was exciting, there was quite a bit of turmoil involved in setting up the new program. Sometimes the faculty members disagreed with Sullivan's decisions. At other times, the medical program's relationship with its parent institution, More-house College, led to additional frustrations. According to David Mann, who was a new faculty member in 1978, "I moved down here from SUNY-Bing-hamton, and within a week, the faculty of the medical school voted 'no con-fidence' in Dean Sullivan."[95] One of the reasons that the 25 faculty members were so upset, according to Mann, was that being part of Morehouse College made the administrative functions of the medical school cumbersome. He recalled: "Since the administrative services were tied to Morehouse College, we had two layers of bureaucracy that you had to go through, for instance when you wanted to purchase things, or if you wanted to get a contract for a secretary. Not only did Lou have to sign off, but also the president of Morehouse College, Hugh Gloster."[96] Some faculty thought that Sullivan wasn't protecting them and their interests in the larger institution.[97]

Unfortunately, other Atlanta University Center administrators did not look on Louis Sullivan as an equal, because his rank was dean, not president. In fact, when the medical school dean's office was moved to Harkness Hall, Atlanta University president Cleveland Dennard would not allow Sullivan to have an office near his own on the second floor, because Sullivan was not a president.[98]

Also, according to Sullivan: "Hugh Gloster was a bit of a micromanager. He had to interview everyone, even secretaries. I told him that I could take care of all matters related to the medical school but Hugh was afraid to fail. He had worked so hard to build Morehouse College and didn't want anything to interfere in its success."[99] Gloster may have had difficulty dealing with Sullivan's personality, as well. According to Gloster's wife, Yvonne, "Hugh was very fond of Lou and considered Lou's hiring one of the best decisions he made as president, but these two men had strong personalities and butted heads once in a while."[100]

The "no confidence" vote by the faculty resulted in an emergency meeting of the executive committee of the Board of Overseers and a hearing in which the faculty aired their complaints. Eventually, one of the board members, Ephraim Friedman, asked President Gloster if he supported the faculty vote.[101] After some ambiguous comments under repeated questioning by Friedman, President Gloster offered his support for Sullivan. The relationship between Dean Sullivan and President Gloster was strained for some time after this incident, but both men moved beyond it, due to their respect for one another. Nonetheless, the problems raised by the faculty and the lack of autonomy allotted to Sullivan accelerated the plan for the medical school to break free of Morehouse College.[102]

Gloster's need to control all aspects of campus life has been well documented by other scholars.[103] While it is possible to view this as the result of one strong-willed individual's ambitions for his institution, it also follows a pattern seen at other Black colleges. Throughout their history, Black college leaders have felt that they were under intense scrutiny by outsiders. Fearing critiques from the surrounding White community—critiques that might lead to decreases in funding from local citizens and foundations, as well as backlash from Black community members—these presidents tended to keep a close watch on their faculty and staff.[104]

Success Overall

Between 1975 and 1980, much was accomplished under Sullivan's leadership. First, the faculty and administration worked to define the program's mission and develop a two-year, basic medical sciences curriculum. Next, Morehouse developed criteria for admissions and made contractual arrangements for transferring students to four-year medical schools—Emory University, the Medical College of Georgia, the University of Alabama at Birmingham, and Howard University—after they completed the basic medical sciences program. Students also transferred to Brown University and the University of Illinois of their own accord.[105] In order to sustain the institution, Sullivan and his staff completed a comprehensive, five-year financial planning effort and initiated fundraising. The administration also established procedures for appointing faculty and staff, and it arranged for space for the medical program in various buildings on the Morehouse College campus.[106]

The charter class of students participated in an "Awards Day" on Friday, June 13, 1980, at which Benjamin E. Mays, mentor to Martin Luther King Jr. and president emeritus of Morehouse College, was the keynote speaker. Mays said to the graduates, "You are now joining an illustrious group of leaders as the first transferring class from the School of Medicine at Morehouse College." Afterwards, he named a long list of distinguished Black Americans who had graduated from Morehouse.[107]

CHAPTER FOUR

Coming into Its Own

Morehouse School of Medicine was incorporated in Georgia on August 12, 1980, with a Board of Overseers that included Calvin Brown, Robert Foreman, Joseph Gayles, Hugh Gloster, Howard Jordan, Nelson McGhee, Louis Sullivan, and Clinton Warner.[1] Sullivan now served as president of the medical school as well as its academic dean. On July 1, 1981, the institution became independent of Morehouse College, and the Board of Overseers became the Board of Trustees. But the medical school received consent from Morehouse College's Board of Trustees to maintain the Morehouse name. The School of Medicine's administration felt that the Morehouse brand would lend them credibility. "Maintaining the Morehouse name really got us off the ground, because of the reputation of the college," said faculty member James Story. "Spelman and Morehouse—not to slight the other colleges in the center, but they were the big-ticket schools. And with Morehouse men having gone into government, everybody that we talked to, almost, had a Morehouse connection. That benefited the school early on."[2]

Sullivan said there were other reasons to maintain the Morehouse name as well: "We didn't have any alumni, people didn't know us, and therefore we really were kind of an unknown entity, whereas everyone knew Morehouse College as a highly respected institution."[3] The medical school administration relied on the Morehouse College alumni quite often during the early years. "If we had a hearing up on Capitol Hill before some congressional committee, we would call on the Morehouse College alumni in Washington to attend that hearing with us," Sullivan said. "Also, at receptions in the D.C. area, the alumni would introduce me to potential funders."[4]

The medical school's use of the Morehouse name also brought advantages to the College. According to sociologists Christopher Jencks and David Riesman, having a medical school affiliation (real or assumed) establishes an institution's "over-all commitment to 'hard,' 'practical' subjects, as against the 'soft,' 'irrelevant' humanities." Moreover, having a medical school affiliated with a private college gives the appearance that an institution is a "public utility" and offsets the notion that colleges and universities are "purely self-serving." Of course, once the legal separation between Morehouse College and Morehouse School of Medicine occurred, all of the benefits became less tangible and based mainly on perception.[5]

After the medical school became independent from Morehouse College in 1981, the president of Atlanta University, Cleveland Dennard, asked Sullivan to make the medical school part of Atlanta University. Dennard saw the immense benefits of having a medical school, including prestige, increased federal funding, and the potential for wealthy alumni.[6] Years had passed since the original discussion of founding a medical school, and Dennard, a relative newcomer, was unaware that Atlanta University had been offered the medical school and rejected it.

When Dennard approached Sullivan, Atlanta University was experiencing hard times. According to Sullivan, medical school administrators knew about Atlanta University's financial problems, and they also questioned whether the institution had the academic strength to support a medical school.[7] And Sullivan hadn't forgotten that Dennard once objected to letting then dean Sullivan have his office on the second floor of Harkness Hall because he was "not a president." Morehouse School of Medicine remained an independent institution.

Breaking Ground on the First Building

In its first six years, Morehouse School of Medicine used makeshift facilities—a major disadvantage to both students and faculty. But with the prodigious fundraising efforts of Sullivan and his staff, the medical school was finally able to construct a building of its own. In April 1980, the School of Medicine broke ground for the Basic Medical Sciences Building, the new institution's first permanent structure. Many well-wishers were on hand, including Governor George Busbee, who told the crowd of dignitaries: "As education has always been one of my top priorities, it is encouraging indeed to see the School of Medicine at Morehouse College successfully open up the area of medical education with a mission of serving the disadvantaged. I am proud to pledge my continued support of this effort."[8]

In 1981, the now independent Morehouse School of Medicine applied for membership in the Atlanta University Center. The new school needed to have the vote of all the other members,[9] and Sullivan visited each of the presidents and boards of trustees of the member institutions to garner their support. The medical school's application was approved unanimously, and it

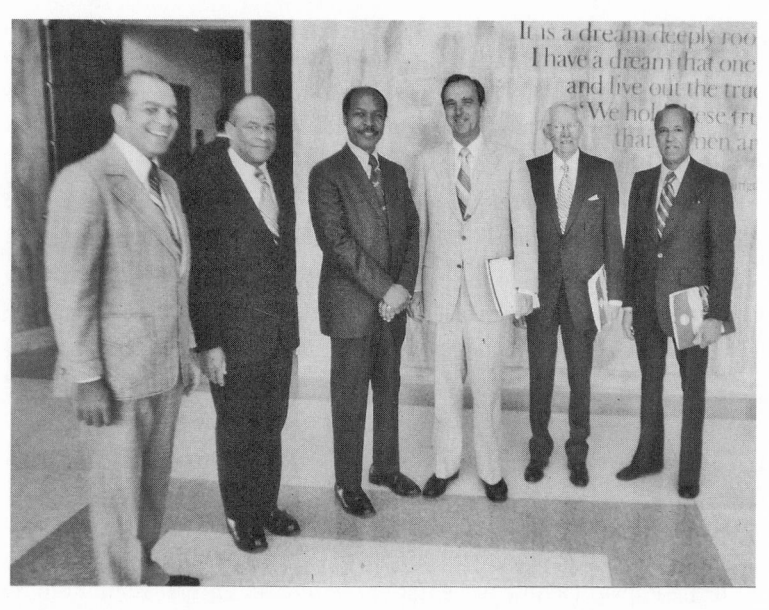

Attendees at the groundbreaking ceremonies for the Basic Medical Sciences Building, April 1980. *Left to right*, President Lloyd Elam of Meharry Medical College, Dean Marion Mann of Howard University School of Medicine, Dean Louis W. Sullivan of the School of Medicine at Morehouse College, Governor of Georgia George Busbee, Chairman of the Fulton County Board of Commissioners Charlie Brown, and President Hugh Gloster of Morehouse College.

became a member on July 1, 1983.[10] Joining the Atlanta University Center let the medical school set up a recruiting pipeline from the Center's colleges and offer research programs across the various colleges.

In 1980, the school established a Transition Campaign Committee to raise money for the transition from an affiliated program in Morehouse College to an independent institution, and from a two-year to a four-year curriculum; community businesses gave almost $2 million. Donald Keough, president of the Coca-Cola Company, who led the campaign, said: "The support received by the Transition Campaign Committee from the Atlanta business community has been excellent. The business leadership in this city is proud of what Morehouse School of Medicine has accomplished in so short a time, and it has backed up that pride with financial support."[11]

Sullivan raised most of the money for the Basic Medical Sciences Building locally. Coca-Cola contributed substantially, and Sullivan worked hand-in-hand with Keough to achieve Morehouse's fundraising goals. Atlanta, according to most locals, is a Coke town. With that in mind, Sullivan recalled a story about his early interactions with Keough:

> About two weeks before the dedication of the Basic Medical Science Building, Don Keough had a luncheon here for the members of the Transition Campaign Committee, to thank them for their work and to introduce them to the building and the school. I got a call from the chief of maintenance saying that Keough had arrived early at the new building. The luncheon was at noon, and he arrived at 11:30 a.m. So I went rushing over to show him around, but he had already walked through the building by the time I got to him. He said, "Lou, you have an interesting building here, and it looks very good. I am very pleased with it, but I ran into a strange vending machine." Well, when he said that, I knew exactly what he had run into—a Pepsi-Cola vending machine. I didn't even know the machine had been placed in the building. But I said, "Don, it will be out before the sun sets," and I called the chief of maintenance and told him to get it out of there![12]

As if the Pepsi machine were not enough of an embarrassment to Sullivan, the choice of wine at the luncheon caused a stir as well. The waiters served bottles of Beringer Chardonnay, wrapped in white cloths. Keough looked up at his waiter and said, "Let me see the label." Unbeknownst to Sullivan, Coca-Cola owned Sterling Vineyards in Napa Valley. The right thing to do when entertaining Keough would have been to select a wine from Sterling. According to Sullivan, Keough said, "Lou, have you ever heard of Sterling wines?" Of course, the answer was no, and Keough asked his assistant, John White, to arrange a visit to Sterling Vineyards the next time Sullivan was in the San Francisco area. "I was so embarrassed," Sullivan said. "We had the wrong vending machine and the wrong wine at an event for our major donor and his committee."[13] Despite the foul-ups, Keough went on to be a generous donor and an avid supporter of the institution. But the flap about the vending machine and the wine illustrates an important characteristic of corporate philanthropy. In the end, corporate donors are interested in advancing their products more than anything else. While the small issues the Coca-Cola president raised were far from the subject of medicine, they were critical to the future success of the medical school.

Attracting Prominence

In 1982, Louis Sullivan's efforts caught the attention of Vice President George H. W. Bush. When President Ronald Reagan declined an invitation to the dedication of the Basic Medical Sciences Building, Sullivan extended one to Vice President Bush.[14] In the end, it was fortuitous that Reagan declined. According to Sullivan: "Reagan had done a couple of things after we had invited him which concerned me to the degree that I said if he accepts and comes, I am going to have to follow him right onto the plane when he leaves. He was not in good standing in the Black community." First, in March 1981, Reagan submitted an education budget that slashed many programs, including those of particular benefit to Black colleges and universities and African Americans in general. For example, at the time financial experts were predicting that African Americans, because of their relatively low incomes, would receive only half as much as Whites in tax cuts as a result of Reagan's budget. On the other hand, Reagan's cuts in housing and education disproportionately hurt Blacks, because 32 percent of Blacks were below the poverty line, compared with only 10 percent of Whites.[15] In other words, Blacks were being asked to pay the same amount of taxes but receive fewer benefits. Then, in August 1981, Reagan expressed support for Bob Jones University in South Carolina, which was fighting to maintain its tax-exempt status in the courts. The religious institution was under scrutiny because it had banned interracial dating on its campus and maintained a segregated campus until 1975.[16] Sullivan admitted that the medical school's administration was trying to figure out a way to withdraw the invitation to Reagan but realized that "you just can't do that." When the president finally turned the school down and sent Vice President Bush instead, the staff members were, in Sullivan's words, "pleased as hell."[17]

Bush's presence was quite a coup for the small campus, drawing attention to Morehouse's accomplishments among the 500 who attended, including many of Atlanta's dignitaries.[18] The dedication provided an occasion to set aside partisan differences. According to Sullivan: "I observed that all of these Black Democratic politicians were fighting to get their picture taken with this Republican vice president: Andy Young, Ed McIntyre (the mayor of Augusta), John Lewis, and all the rest. So that really was the nature of the excitement we had in having the vice president of the United States here for the ribbon-cutting for our first building."[19]

The dedication of the Basic Medical Sciences Building was especially significant in the history of Morehouse School of Medicine, because prior to that time the school was operating on the Morehouse College campus and was scattered all around that institution. If anyone came looking for Morehouse School of Medicine, they could barely find evidence of its existence unless

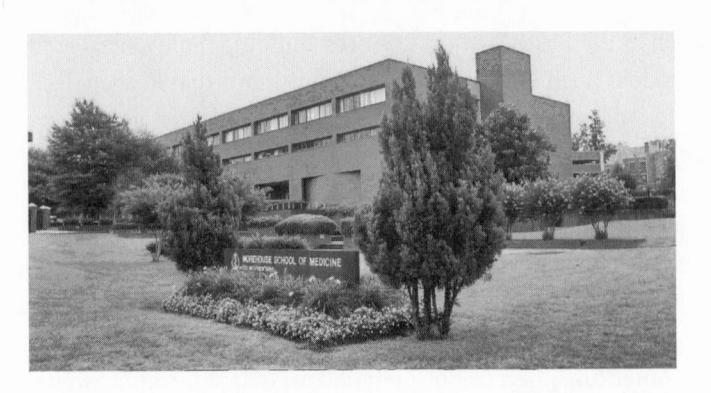

The completed Basic Medical Sciences Building.

they stumbled into a classroom—or a cadaver—because the institution was merely occupying temporary facilities on the Morehouse College campus.[20]

As a result of their meeting, Sullivan and Bush became friends. Soon after, Bush invited Sullivan to accompany him on a two-week tour of African countries in November 1982—the first high-profile visit to Sub-Saharan Africa by a senior member of Reagan's administration. The purpose of the visit was to "broaden communications and understanding between the United States and its people and the nations of Africa and their people."[21] According to Sullivan, "the vice president felt that a Black American leader who was not a government official would add credibility to the delegation among the African nations."[22] Sullivan also befriended first lady Barbara Bush on this trip, and he won her participation on the medical school's Board of Trustees. Because of these top-echelon associations, Sullivan began to be seen as a national leader on issues related to medical education for minorities. Still, he had much to do in terms of expanding the medical school.[23]

From a Two-Year to a Four-Year Institution

Although Morehouse School of Medicine had successful transfer programs with Emory University, the Medical College of Georgia, Howard University, and the University of Alabama at Birmingham, the institution's long-range plan had always been to develop into a four-year medical school. According to Charles Stephens, the institution's first fundraiser: "One of the biggest challenges ahead of us was that we were in a situation where we weren't taking the students from beginning to end. We had to develop liaison relationships with other medical schools that would be comfortable taking our

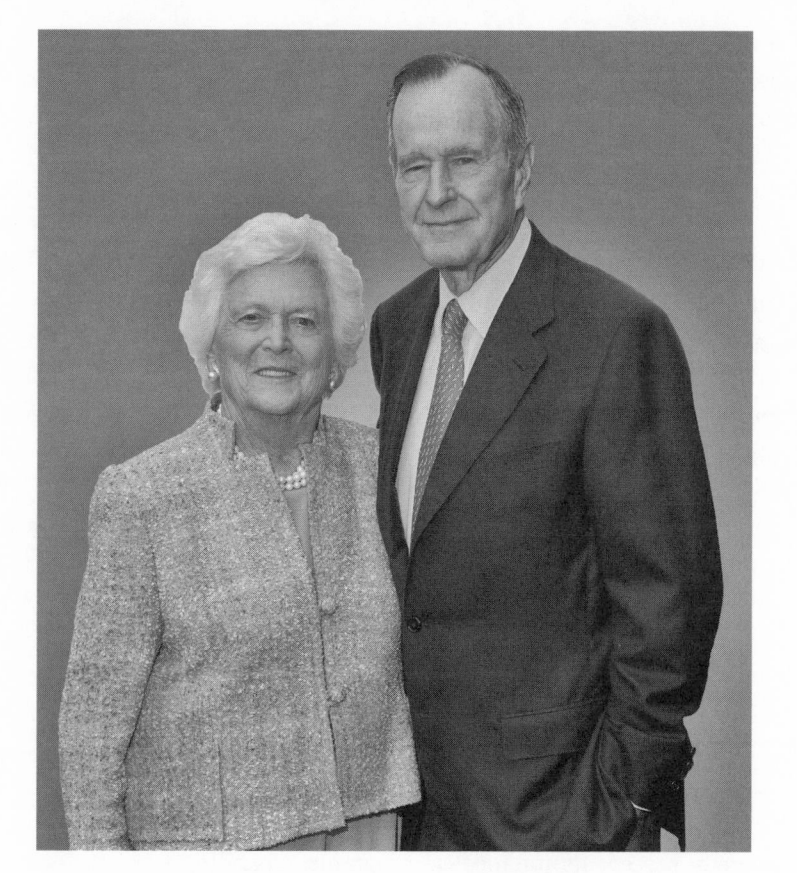

President George H. W. Bush and Barbara Bush.

students after two years. This was a huge barrier to overcome."[24] Moreover, because Morehouse's alumni during that time received their MDs from another institution, they had split loyalties.

In the early 1980s, health care costs were rising, medical malpractice insurance rates were soaring, and there was constant public scrutiny of the medical profession.[25] It was in this climate that Morehouse School of Medicine became a four-year program. One ally in this effort was Emory Medical Center CEO Charles Hatcher. Like Sullivan, Hatcher was from rural southwest Georgia. He attended the Medical College of Georgia and did his residency with the pioneer heart surgeon Alfred Blalock, working closely with Blalock's African American assistant, Vivien Thomas. Blalock and Thomas became famous for their work on blue baby syndrome; Thomas eventually gained recognition for his contributions despite being unable to attend medical school because of racial discrimination and a lack of finances. Hatcher's experience with Thomas made him sympathetic to Morehouse School of Medicine and its mission. In many ways, Thomas exemplified the reasons why Morehouse School of Medicine was needed.

Before Morehouse School of Medicine became a four-year program, Hatcher ensured that Emory was willing to accept third- and fourth-year students from the institution into its medical program, as long as the students passed the national board exams.[26] When the time came, Hatcher gave Sullivan advice on how to move the program to the next level. According to Hatcher: "The problem was that they had a two-year school, and accrediting agencies at that time had determined in their wisdom that there weren't going to be any more two-year schools. You had to either close or become a four-year school."[27]

During the early years, Morehouse had a contract with Emory for access to its clinical faculty. This contract lasted for six years, but when it came time to renew it for a second term, Hatcher became uneasy. According to the Emory CEO, "I thought that if this relationship continued too long, Morehouse would develop a hostile dependency on Emory."[28] Hatcher suggested that Morehouse instead go forward and become a four-year institution. He told Sullivan to plunge right in and offer the last two years of the medical program on the Morehouse campus, assuring him that Emory would provide the professors if the Black medical school ran short.[29] In fact, there were numerous precedents for medical programs expanding from two to four years,[30] including those at Dartmouth College, the University of Mississippi, the University of Nevada, and the University of North Carolina.[31]

The AMA joined Hatcher in advising Morehouse to expand. In 1982, James H. Sammons, the executive vice president of the AMA, visited the institution and was impressed with what he saw. Sammons expressed confidence that Morehouse was ready to forge ahead with its desire to become a four-year medical school—in spite of the difficult climate many medical schools faced at the time. He pointed out that "some very old, staid schools, both public and private, may be forced to close their doors."[32] Yet Sammons saw a great need for Morehouse and its unique program, noting the special role predominantly Black institutions played in medical education. Sammons was able to see the niche that Morehouse filled—that of educating students of color, those who wanted to focus on medicine in poor urban and rural areas, and those interested in primary care.[33] He was also impressed that the Georgia legislature had recognized Morehouse's work and was ap-

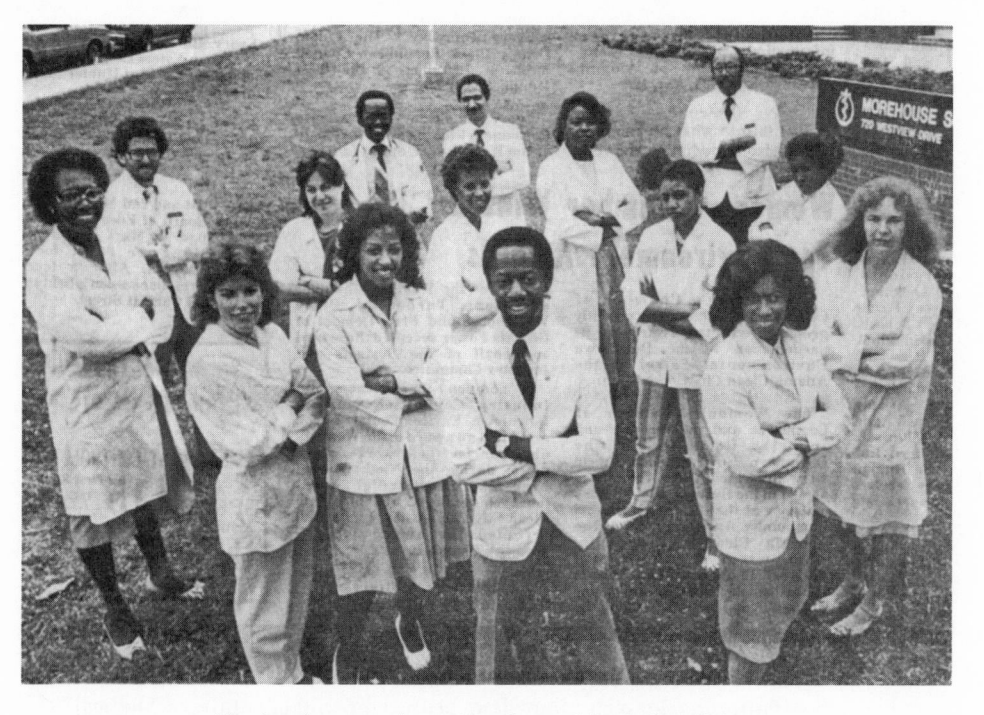

The first four-year class at Morehouse School of Medicine.

propriating state funds to the institution. Although he acknowledged that some parts of the country had too many doctors, Sammons noted that the "sunbelt" states were in dire need of physicians.[34]

As Sammons's accreditation visit took place, the Institute of Medicine in Washington, D.C., was conducting a major review of medical education. In 1983, they issued an influential report, *Medical Education and Societal Needs: A Planning Report for the Health Professions,* which called for the medical school curriculum to have a better connection with societal concerns and issues of social justice.[35] Unlike many medical schools across the country that had strayed from their original missions of training doctors toward a heavy research agenda, or moved from creating primary care doctors to medical specialists, Morehouse had put issues of social justice and primary care at its core.

Administrative Restructuring amid Change

As the change from two-year to four-year status moved forward, Morehouse also restructured its leadership. In 1983 the positions of dean and president were separated, because it became obvious to Sullivan and the Board of Trustees that the responsibilities of each of these positions demanded a full-time person.[36] The dean presided over the faculty, curriculum, and students; the president represented the institution to the outside world, raised funds, helped to recruit administrative staff, and worked with the trustees and donors.

Stanley Olson served as the first dean after Sullivan. In a sign of the medical school's interest in diversity from its inception, Olson was White. He was an ideal choice, because he had been involved in the two-year to four-year transition from an early date. In 1977 and 1978, he served as a consultant, writing a plan that would ultimately be used for the transition.

When Morehouse initiated its four-year program, it had to develop an affiliation with a teaching hospital where students would be placed for the second half of the program, which would focus on clinical training. Grady Memorial Hospital, a distinguished teaching facility in the center of Atlanta, boasted a mission in line with that of Morehouse. Grady is a large county hospital whose users include a substantial proportion of poor and minority patients. According to Emory's Charles Hatcher, Grady had "taken care of the black population as long as there had been a hospital."[37] Emory Medical School used Grady as its clinical site, but Emory faculty initially hesitated at the idea of sharing the facility with Morehouse. According to Emory Assistant Dean Jonas Shulman, their faculty were aware that such an arrangement could be difficult. They knew, for example, that Philadelphia General Hospital had tried and failed to operate in conjunction with four medical schools, and that Boston City Hospital had not succeeded in its attempt to accommodate the medical schools at Harvard, Boston, and Tufts Universities. Eventually, after extensive negotiation and competition, only Boston University used Boston City Hospital as its clinical site. These experiences in other cities made some Emory faculty worry about the future of the Grady-Emory-Morehouse partnership.[38]

But Louis Sullivan and Charles Hatcher were determined to forge a productive relationship that would benefit all partners. Hatcher commented:

> Now, you can understand that not every doctor who had spent his career at Grady was happy with another medical school coming in. Two medical schools using the same public facility sometimes causes difficulty, and Morehouse was a new school and Emory was a very old school. Some people thought there might be a difference in the level of expertise that would be unacceptable, but I made the decision that we

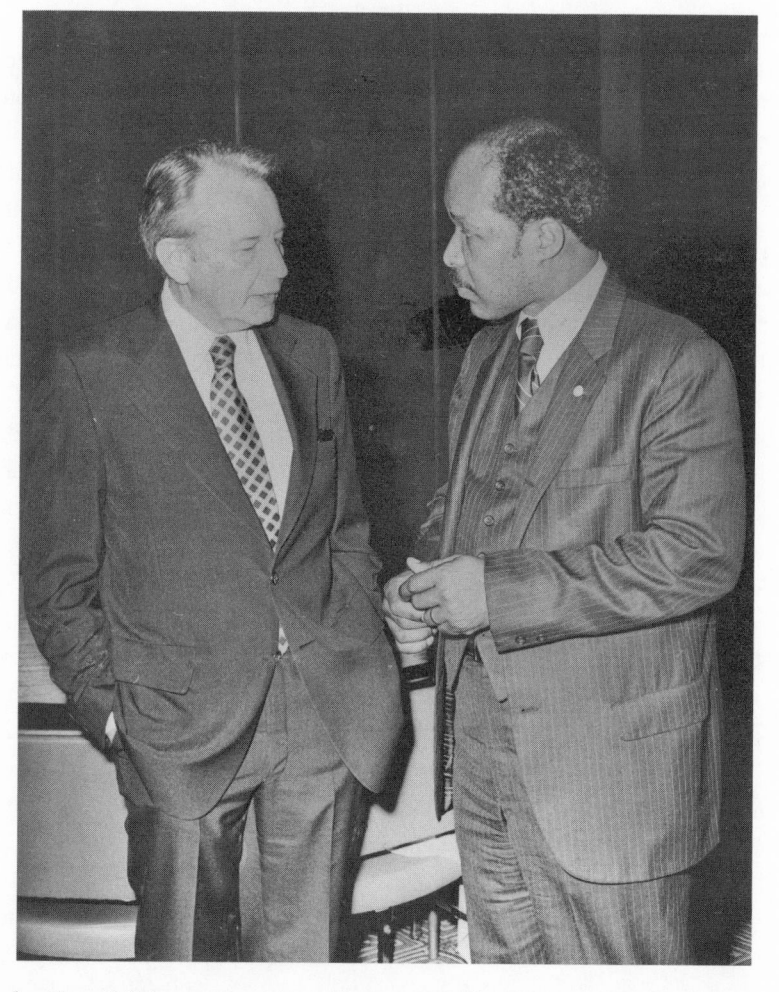

Stanley Olson (*left*) in a conversation with Louis W. Sullivan (*right*). Photograph courtesy of Roland Welmaker.

were going to amend our contract, we'd give Morehouse access, and negotiate what was the proper amount of responsibility for Morehouse to assume without overburdening itself.[39]

Hatcher knew how much time and effort it took to make Grady a teaching environment that was satisfactory to Emory; with regard to Morehouse, he could see that taking on too much of Grady at one time might burden the new institution, financially and otherwise. According to Hatcher, one of the reasons the negotiations with Morehouse went so smoothly was that the institution had immense respect for Sullivan. Emory had tried to recruit Sullivan as a hematologist when he finished training in Boston. In Hatcher's words: "You're always better off if you're working from a position of professional admiration for the person that you're negotiating with. So there was no question that Emory held him in high esteem, and I personally held him in high esteem, so we worked this out."

Hatcher and Sullivan agreed to ground rules. First, they decided not to say anything negative about the Morehouse-Emory relationship and refused to be "drawn into a critical situation in the press."[40] Second, they met regularly and spoke frankly. If there was a problem that needed attention, they handled it internally. According to Hatcher, "we worked it out between the two of us, behind closed doors." Lastly, Sullivan and Hatcher crafted a process to deal with disagreements among the Emory and Morehouse faculty. As Hatcher describes it: "If somebody's feelings were hurt or somebody didn't think they were being treated fairly, then we would not wait until that came up the next month at some regular meeting. We would address that right away. I believe in lancing a boil before it gets to be too big, and if someone had a complaint, let's let Lou and me hear it and solve it and go on to the next thing." Asa Yancey Sr., an African American physician who was the chief medical officer at Grady Hospital and was on the faculty at Emory University, said the reason the Morehouse-Grady relationship worked was that "the people in charge wanted it to work, and they just made it clear it's going to work. And that attitude filters down from the top to everyone."[41]

Grady Memorial Hospital had a national reputation as a training institution and a long legacy in the Atlanta area. Initially it had served both Blacks and Whites, but by the late 1960s the patients were about 95 percent African American. In Hatcher's mind, having Morehouse use the hospital for its clinical teaching made sense. When some Emory faculty didn't want to "share" the facility with Morehouse, he pushed back, proclaiming, "Do you think I'm going to stand in the hospital door like George Wallace and say 'You can't have anything to do with all of these Black patients!' when you have a Black hospital board, a Black mayor, a Black city council, a predominantly Black hospital authority? You have to make accommodations."[42]

Due to past racial tensions, Atlanta's public hospital authority was also skeptical. When Hatcher and Sullivan brought their plan to the hospital authority, the response was, "I can tell you right now we're not going to sign off on anything about the hospital until there's a satisfactory agreement between Morehouse and Emory." Sullivan and Hatcher emphasized that the two schools had in fact reached an agreement. But the cautious hospital authority, which included many prominent African Americans who had weathered the racial storms in Georgia, couldn't quite imagine it. According to Hatcher, "it was almost like they couldn't believe that we had reached an agreement between the Black and White schools."[43]

Even some Morehouse people had difficulty understanding how an agreement between the two schools could be reached in such an amicable way. They doubted Emory's sincerity and its willingness to act in Morehouse's best interest. Clinton Warner, the chair of Morehouse School of Medicine's board at the time, was concerned that all of the money associated with the program was deposited in Emory's accounts and never came directly to Morehouse. Warner had seen such agreements in the past and argued that they typically worked to the detriment of the smaller institution. He cautioned Sullivan against jumping into the agreement. Despite Warner's misgivings, Sullivan moved forward, and in the end the agreement was a sign of how Atlanta's racial climate had improved.[44]

Even with a well-crafted agreement between the schools, Hatcher and Sullivan could not predict how students from the very different institutions would interact. From time to time, Emory students working at Grady expressed the belief that Morehouse students were not of the same quality. Sullivan worked to counter these ideas by bringing in the best class of students possible and implementing special support programs to amply prepare them for their Grady Hospital experience.[45] Hatcher also noticed the tension. "I think it's natural for anyone to have a little turf feeling when you're first getting started," he said, "but we were very careful to have as little arbitrary action as we could."[46] For example, Hatcher insisted that the two schools have an equitable system for receiving patients in the emergency room. He told the hospital administration that they needed to work out a numbers system— every fourth patient would go to Morehouse, for instance. He did not want Emory to be accused of picking the most interesting patients or working only with the paying patients. The system had to be random, and Hatcher asked that it be controlled by him and Sullivan.[47]

A curious result of the embedded bias of the times was that sometimes a White physician would pay a Morehouse student a backhanded compliment. Gary MaGaha, Sullivan's presidential assistant during the early years, recalled a few occasions when some of the White Morehouse students were mistaken for Emory students. White physicians would say: "You Emory students are really talented. We like what you are doing. Keep up the good job."

And the White Morehouse student would respond: "Well, actually, I am a Morehouse student who just happens to be White. Morehouse is integrated." MaGaha kept track of these comments, and he and President Sullivan worked to counter the notion that Morehouse was for Black students only.[48]

Fully Accredited

The rules of the Liaison Committee on Medical Education stated that new medical schools were not eligible to receive full accreditation until they offered all four years of the curriculum. Morehouse School of Medicine reached this milestone in April 1985, and its first class of MDs graduated that year from a fully accredited medical school.[49] The first commencement was held on May 17, 1985, and 21 MD degrees were awarded. On the day the school received news of the accreditation, President Sullivan noted that "we have come from three or four people in a trailer with an idea to a fully developed, fully accredited institution with 154 people on the payroll and 122 students."[50] Cyril Moore, then chairman of the Department of Biochemistry, said: "There were many who thought we would never make it. There's a need, a purpose for this school. You can feel it in your bones."[51] Sullivan's further comment that day was interesting, and telling, given the political context of the times: the school was "not simply a good Black medical school, but a good medical school that happens to be Black."[52]

Beginning in late 1986, the medical school took on the responsibility of staffing and operating Hughes Spalding Medical Center, an affiliate of the Fulton-DeKalb Hospital Authority, as well as Southwest Hospital, which is a small hospital owned and operated by African Americans in the heart of a Black, middle-class community. Both facilities provided a place to house the Morehouse faculty's medical practice plan, but they lacked the infrastructure to serve as teaching hospitals.

New Funding Sources

Having full accreditation made it much easier to garner funds from potential donors. In 1987 Morehouse School of Medicine received a $225,000 contribution from the Health 1st Foundation, an affiliate of Health 1st, the first health maintenance organization in Atlanta. Health 1st was founded in 1975 by four local Black physicians—Clinton Warner, Delutha King, Nelson Mc-Ghee, and Andrew Randolph. When Delutha King presented the check to

Clinton Warner, who by then was chair of the Morehouse medical school's board, Warner said:

> It is equally appropriate that I, as chairman of the board of Morehouse School of Medicine and one of the founders of Health 1st, should be present on this occasion to receive the first installment of $60,000. I am also proud of the participation and founding of Health 1st by Black physicians in Atlanta. There could be no better purpose for the contribution than to assist Morehouse School of Medicine in its efforts to endow our faculty development at Grady Memorial Hospital. Until the medical school has developed fully its clinical faculty and reached a stable level of financial support from its hospital affiliations and its faculty practice plan . . . contributions such as this one make a major difference in our meeting our objective on a timely basis.[53]

Although U.S. medical schools went through a period of retrenchment after a 1977 report by the Graduate Medical Education National Advisory Committee said that there were too many physicians, Morehouse School of Medicine nonetheless flourished because of the need for Black physicians and for primary care physicians in medically underserved areas. In 1988, for example, despite a surplus of doctors in general, less than 3.2 percent of U.S. physicians were African American, and more than 30 million Americans lived in areas officially designated as medically underserved.[54]

Morehouse School of Medicine also benefited from its willingness to reach out to other countries that were in dire need of primary medical care. In 1987, under Sullivan's direction, the school began work to help alleviate health care problems in Liberia, Nigeria, Zimbabwe, and Senegal. During Sullivan's 1982 visit to Africa with Vice President Bush, he saw first hand that "diseases that have been virtually eliminated in the U.S. were still killing Africans."[55] The medical school president wanted to be out in front when it came to working across international borders to increase access to health care, and he secured ample support for the school's efforts. For example, the U.S. Agency for International Development gave Morehouse School of Medicine money to train primary care doctors and traditional healers in Senegal and operate HIV/AIDS programs in Zambia, Lesotho, and Swaziland.

In 1987, state senator Horace E. Tate, well known for his role in merging the Black and White teacher associations in Georgia, helped the medical school acquire $5 million from the Georgia budget. He benefited from the help of longtime state representative Calvin Smyre and Governor Joe Frank Harris, who were known for their support of educational initiatives in the state.[56] When Harris became governor of Georgia in 1983, the medical school started to receive more regular allotments from the state. Harris was impressed with the school's mission of educating primary care physicians and reaching out to underserved and low-income populations.[57] Not everyone in Georgia, however, appreciated the state's funding of Morehouse School of Medicine. In May 1989 Jasper Dorsey, an op-ed writer for the *Athens Metropolitan Area* newspaper, wrote: "The Medical College of Georgia is of excellent quality but that could be raised if the millions of tax money wasn't spent supporting medical schools at two private colleges, Mercer and Morehouse [Mercer ultimately got its medical school]. Tax support for a church school and a private school is not good policy, especially when we have a glut of physicians."[58] Of course, Dorsey did not consider the dire need for African American physicians and those who were willing to work in primary care and in low-income communities.

In 1987 the medical school also received a $2 million grant, shepherded by Sullivan, from the Robert Wood Johnson Foundation—at the time, the largest private grant in the school's history. With this influx of funding, the medical school was definitely coming into its own as an institution.[59] And as one of three predominantly Black medical schools in the nation, Morehouse was poised to receive the attention of foundations with a commitment to social justice and to assisting those with little access to quality health care.[60]

Morehouse Gains a Top Fundraiser

As we've noted, Louis Sullivan and Barbara Bush became fast friends after they met during Vice President Bush's two-week visit to Africa in November 1982. During the trip, Sullivan invited Mrs. Bush to serve on Morehouse's Board of Trustees, and she agreed. "He persuaded me, and I'm still persuaded, that minorities, rural and urban, are underserved," Mrs. Bush said. "The medical school has been relatively successful at training doctors— young men and women—to work in rural communities and urban areas."[61] Mrs. Bush was also moved to participate, in part, because of her daughter Robin's death from leukemia; she cared deeply about access to proper medical care. By her own admission, she knew little about medical education or services for minorities or the poor until she started working with Morehouse School of Medicine. She said: "Before Lou explained the mission of the school to me, I had never really thought about it. I lived a sheltered life. Something about the mission of the school resonated with me, however."[62] Sullivan's close tie to Barbara Bush helped raise the public image of Morehouse School of Medicine. The school now had access to high-profile venues.[63] For example, when New York Yankees outfielder Dave M. Winfield agreed to be on the Morehouse School of Medicine board in 1987, George and Barbara Bush held the announcement ceremony at the Vice President's residence.[64]

Mrs. Bush began serving in January 1983, and she spearheaded a $15 million fundraising campaign for the school.[65] As a result, many corporate leaders paid attention to Morehouse School of Medicine. For instance, Stanley Pace, the chief executive of General Dynamics, hosted his own fundraiser for Morehouse in St. Louis, Missouri, after being introduced to the school by Barbara Bush; he donated $250,000 of his own money to the institution. Of note, a defense contractor like General Dynamics would most likely not have been interested in the cause of Black medicine were it not for the influence of the Bushes.

The first lady traveled the country with Sullivan, raising money for the medical school. As she recalled:

> It was hard. They had no alumni, and so occasionally we'd find one and we'd come and testify, and he or she would be working in the field that we were hoping they would be. By that I mean that we hoped they would go back to rural neighborhoods where nobody was served or to inner cities. Most young doctors want to go where the money is, but these young people were trained to go back and serve rural and urban communities. As I recall, about 80 percent were committed to the school's mission in this way.[66]

Mrs. Bush and Sullivan met with CEOs of companies in cities across the country. "We raised money because Lou Sullivan does not accept no," she said. "I mean, he would even want to come and see us [the Bushes], and we'd say, 'We can't see you,' and he'd ask, 'Why not?' And we'd say, 'Because we're going to say no to your request.' And then he'd come anyway, and we'd end up saying yes to him."[67]

Mrs. Bush was a very active board member who "enjoyed the board meetings." In particular, she rose to the challenge of organizing high-profile fundraising activities. "We would plan grand and expensive events," she said, "and Lou could always get the support for them." She recalled one board meeting in particular, when she learned that the medical school had recently gained accreditation. She had been serving for two years and was shocked that the institution was just now being accredited. She joked with Sullivan: "You mean we weren't accredited all these years and I've been out there raising money?" Of course, Sullivan explained that the school had provisional accreditation for years before it offered a four-year curriculum. Mrs. Bush said: "In a very brief time for a medical school, he got this school accredited, and it's pretty hard not to have huge respect for a man who brought the institution from trailers to the school it is today." Mrs. Bush also recognized Sullivan's knack for bipartisanship. "Lou was smart enough not to be political," she said. "He went both ways—Democrat and Republican—as far as seeking aid and help. For instance, Jimmy Carter helped the institution as well as us."[68]

President Sullivan Is Tapped for National Service

President Sullivan maintained a good relationship with both Bushes. President George H. W. Bush said that the relationship was "very personal and very pleasant and [one of] great respect on my part."[69] In November 1988, when Bush won the presidential election, he tapped Louis Sullivan to be the U.S. Secretary of Health and Human Services. As with the Morehouse position, Sullivan first recommended someone else, only to be offered the position himself. During the 1988 state primary elections, Sullivan had suggested to then candidate Bush that the position be filled by one of Morehouse School of Medicine's trustees. Bush agreed to review Sullivan's choice if he won the presidency.[70]

The day after the election, Sullivan called the president-elect to congratulate him and to remind him to consider the Morehouse trustee. President Bush told Sullivan that he had circulated the name around his transition team and it was not getting the response that he needed to take the person forward for confirmation. He asked Sullivan if he would come to Washington in about two weeks to discuss the matter further. Sullivan agreed. But based on his previous experience with such invitations, he had a sneaking suspicion that something else was afoot.

Sure enough, when he traveled to the White House, he figured out exactly who Bush wanted as secretary. According to Sullivan, "the newspapers were smarter than I was because when I got to the White House there were reporters outside, including reporters from the *Atlanta Journal-Constitution*, wanting to know if I had a meeting with the president-elect that morning and, if so, what was it all about."[71] Bush offered Sullivan the position that day. The medical school president was flattered but had mixed emotions: "I didn't feel as if I had finished the job that I was really doing in developing this new medical school."[72] According to President Bush: "I was looking around for a guy who was knowledgeable in the medical field and of course Lou had great credentials. It didn't hurt that he was a minority. In fact, I think that was an asset—a strong asset. I also needed someone who could run a huge department. Though Lou didn't have a lot of management experience, he just impressed me as somebody who could make tough decisions, and he did."[73]

Sullivan's move to Washington caused a controversy at Morehouse School of Medicine. During his 13–year tenure as president of the medical school, Sullivan had never taken a sabbatical. When he left, he asked the board to compensate him in lieu of his earned sabbatical time.[74] Clinton Warner, then chairman of the board, opposed Sullivan's request because he believed it violated federal policies.[75] A meeting of the board's executive committee was called, hosted by Barbara Bush, in the upstairs living quarters of the White House. The White House counsel advised that Sullivan's request did not violate any federal policies. Consequently, the Executive Committee of Morehouse School of Medicine formally voted to honor it. Although this policy matter was resolved, the rift between Warner and Sullivan remained,[76] signaling the start of a rocky period for the institution.

CHAPTER FIVE

Leadership in Transition

It had been many years since Louis Sullivan's first term as president began in 1981. With the founder and robust leader of the institution leaving to take another position in 1989, what would become of Morehouse School of Medicine? In many respects, the institution maintained the course that Sullivan had set for it. But the period of steady growth that ensued in that year also showed that Morehouse was able to flourish on its own—and, when the time came, the institution would be able to cut loose from its moorings and move forward without the founder's leadership.

Steady and Measured Leadership

When Louis Sullivan left to become U.S. Secretary of Health and Human Services under President George H. W. Bush in 1989, the Board of Trustees picked James Goodman to lead Morehouse School of Medicine. Goodman had been executive vice president of the medical school for four years, was an alumnus of Morehouse College, and was a personal friend of Sullivan's.[1] Unlike Sullivan, he held a PhD rather than an MD, and this worried a few of the faculty, who wondered whether an academic, rather than a health professional, was the right choice for president of a medical school.[2] Around the country, faculty members at other medical schools had similar concerns: could a person whose experience was mainly in academic research rather than clinical practice lead an institution for the training of doctors?[3] However, the concerns did not last long at Morehouse. Goodman, who had joined Morehouse School of Medicine in 1980 as the associate dean for administration, was promoted to vice president for administration and policy and in 1985 became the executive vice president.[4] He was a familiar and trusted face at the medical school.

Goodman graduated from Morehouse College in 1956 and earned a master's degree in social work from Atlanta University in 1958. He eventually received a PhD in social work and sociology from the University of Minnesota. His background included extensive experience in both field- and class-

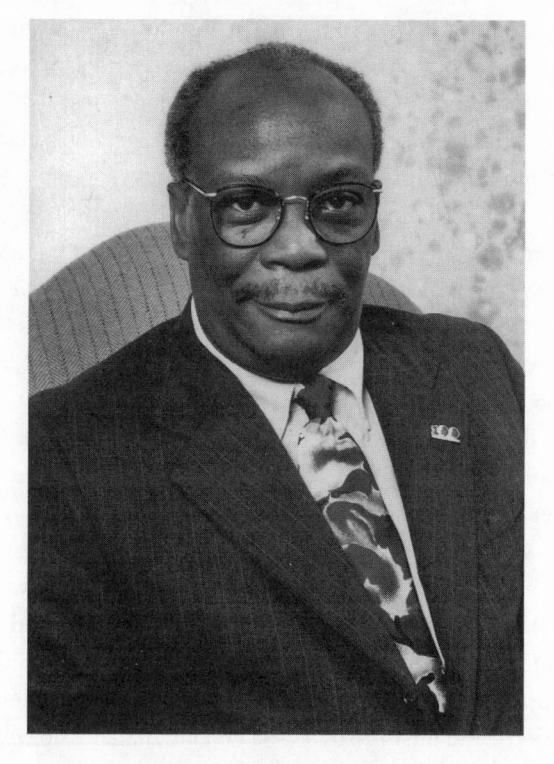

James Goodman, PhD.

room-based social work. He had ample administrative experience, having worked at the U.S. Department of State as the director of the Office of International Training throughout the 1970s. In this position, he planned educational activities between foreign governments and the United States.[5]

Clinton Warner was the chair of the Morehouse Board of Trustees when Goodman was named president. According to Warner, the small medical school did not have the "luxury of conducting a nationwide search for a new president and reviewed fewer than a dozen applications." He noted that Goodman had strong ties to the medical school and that these would be essential during a time of transition: "As a new, developing school, we built up momentum, and we did not want to allow that momentum to slow down. Institutional memory is preserved by selecting a qualified person from the inside."[6]

At the time of the transition, Morehouse's leadership thought the institution was on an even keel, but observers at competing institutions saw the situation differently. For example, Russell L. Miller, the vice president of health affairs at Howard University in Washington, D.C., said that "it does not have the endowment or the funds some other schools have; also, it does not have the reputation."[7] Of course, this comment most likely indicated a sense of competition between the two Black medical schools and the fact that Morehouse was a newer institution.

Goodman had no ambitions to replace Sullivan. In fact, he had just purchased a Jiffy Lube franchise in Seattle and was planning to move there when he was asked to lead the medical school. A recent column in the *New York Times* had even discussed Goodman's plans to manage the franchise. Just as Louis Sullivan was being tapped to be Secretary of Health and Human Services, he saw the article about Goodman's departure in the *Times* and said: "You can't go. I need you here." Despite his plan to move to Seattle, and with the full support of the Board of Trustees, Goodman accepted Morehouse's offer of the presidency.

The former executive vice president was a logical choice. He had good relationships with the faculty and staff, and he had filled presidential functions during Sullivan's administration. When Sullivan was away from campus raising money to sustain the institution, he had entrusted Goodman to manage the medical school's daily operations.[8] According to Sullivan, Goodman "maintained a steady ship; he wasn't a charismatic leader. Instead, he was quiet, serious, and businesslike"[9]—a good manager who was particularly skilled at handling the budget and recruiting strong staff members to ensure continuity.[10] Goodman described himself similarly as "fair but firm," a "good organizer and highly focused."[11] The faculty had confidence in his decisions, because he expressed clear reasoning for them. He did not tolerate nonsense, and he held people accountable for their actions, raising questions when necessary and preferring to discuss issues rather than personalities. Goodman was also highly disciplined about his own work, although relaxed in his manner. According to Gary MaGaha, who stayed on as special assistant to the president when Sullivan left for Washington, President Goodman was "much more laid back" than Sullivan. He added, "Jim was a very confident and capable administrator, but he did not have the fervor for this that Sullivan had."[12] In his own words, Goodman was not the type of leader who drew attention to himself, but rather someone who led by motivating others. He believed that if he set the right example and held high expectations, others would follow through and take the initiative to build the institution. Rather than take credit for the institution's accomplishments, he gave credit to the team.[13] This approach helped to maintain a positive atmosphere at Morehouse during his presidency.[14]

Although some members of the medical school community wondered how the new president would fill Sullivan's shoes, Goodman felt confident about his own leadership. As he described it, Sullivan was "more focused on immediate outcomes, with a sense of what he wanted long term." Goodman did many of the same things he had done under Sullivan's leadership, maintaining a consistent direction in the institution's day-to-day activities.[15] The secret to his success, he said, was that "I'm as apolitical as they come. I don't carry anything around that is a secret. I don't want anyone to help me get an empire going. I've lived the same way wherever I've been—what you see is what you get."[16]

As we've noted, during the civil rights era, and even as early as the post–Civil War Reconstruction era, opponents of racial progress would often spread the rumor that outsiders were coming in to tamper with the Southern way of life.[17] Goodman, in fact, did not hail from the South and might have been vulnerable to such accusations were it not for his talent for communication and diplomacy.[18] He spent time learning where people stood politically. For example, when speaking to a White rural Georgian, he might mention his family's working-class background: "Well, my daddy used to work in a place just like this. I'm sure he would have gotten along with you very well." Goodman fully understood the importance of social connections:

> In the South, people operate on a personal level. It's who you know, who knows you, and what they think of you and how long you've been there, either in a personal sense or in a historical sense—for instance, your parents lived there. Those are the important ingredients in Southern relationships. And once you understand that, you begin to use it in a positive way, to say, "Look, I've been here long enough to know what the protocols are, and I'm not going to abuse them." Once those are understood, there comes about a transformation of the impossible. You are no longer an outsider.[19]

During his administration, Goodman embarked on an effort to eliminate any remnants of the idea that Morehouse, as a historically Black institution, was a transplant from the outside. He helped rally members of the local community, including business people and doctors, to support the medical school. He continued Sullivan's efforts to make sure the institution's funding was a local affair, rather than relying exclusively on outside philanthropy. "We wanted the community to take ownership of the institution," Goodman said. "We couldn't impose the medical school on the community; instead, we needed the community with us on all aspects of our work and development. They need to say, 'This is my medical school.' "[20]

Goodman's political savvy paid off, earning him strong connections with Atlanta locals.[21] He spoke everywhere on behalf of the school. As he describes it, he couldn't keep up with the demand for him as a speaker from both the Black and White communities.[22] These opportunities to get in front of the various audiences in Atlanta helped the school expand its reach and enhance the significance of the work it was doing.[23] One issue that Goodman felt quite strongly about was the school's relationship with Black doctors in Atlanta. This group was concerned that the medical school might take away some of its patients—who were an individual doctor's livelihood. To counter this fear, Goodman made sure that local Black doctors were eligible to participate in the Morehouse School of Medicine practice plan. As noted earlier, the medical school also built a clinic on the campus of Southwest Community Hospital, located in the Black community near the school. Black doctors benefited from this arrangement because it enabled them to mentor Morehouse students and participate in conferences. Moreover, the hospital gave them office space.[24]

Under Goodman's leadership in the late 1980s and early 1990s, the medical school was at the forefront of providing HIV/AIDS education in the African American community. Morehouse offered school-based workshops that highlighted the causes and prevention strategies using startling photographs and statistics, making an effort to motivate young people to practice safe habits. In many instances the medical school would partner with community organizations, such as the African American women's social service group, the Links, to deliver HIV/AIDS education.[25]

Goodman made good use of his connections to further the medical school's interests. In 1990, he was appointed to the International Olympic Committee's Medical Commission for a six-year term. In this capacity, the Morehouse president helped the school land the responsibility of running the drug testing program for the 1996 Olympic Games.[26] As a result, the Atlanta Olympic Committee built a small laboratory building on the Morehouse School of Medicine campus, which, after the Olympics, was developed into a research facility for the school. It now houses the ambulatory research unit, the Neuroscience Research Institute, and other medical research laboratories.

Because Goodman felt strongly about primary care, he extended the institution's focus in this area. He traveled the state to find residencies that gave students practical experience in primary care. According to Goodman, many of the clinical sites were in communities that received little medical attention and "had never seen a medical school come in and do this kind of work."[27]

Goodman was particularly proud of securing reaccreditation for the medical school from the Liaison Committee on Medical Education and the Southern Association of Colleges and Schools. Because the accreditation team leader was the provost at the University of Mississippi, Goodman was worried about the outcome. Ole Miss had a sordid reputation for its treatment of African American students. When the Mississippi provost "walked in with that southern drawl and that gangly walk," the Morehouse president expected the worst. But when the provost opened his mouth to speak, the words that came out were, "Well, I've been looking around here, and it looks pretty good." The medical school not only received full reaccreditation, it was given commendations for its approach to problem solving and its high degree of preparation for the accreditation team's visit.[28] Interestingly, Goodman came to count the Mississippi provost among his friends, and as a strong ally of the medical school. According to Goodman: "You don't build relationships for the moment when leading an institution. You build them to sustain the institution, and they should outlive your term as leader."

Student enrollment flourished under President Goodman. In fact, the medical school had more applicants than it could handle. According to Goodman, "the real issue was making sure that [we] had a class of students that was competent." He wanted students who could successfully take exams and move through the program efficiently and effectively—students who "would not be a drag on the system." In Goodman's words:

> This is important for any institution, but minority-serving institutions are under heightened scrutiny to meet all of the requirements of accreditation and more. We had to make sure our students could compete, so we built in structures such as interactive libraries and support systems that were available day and night to them. We wanted to give the students a leg up.[29]

Since their creation, Black colleges have had a difficult relationship with accrediting organizations, and, as Goodman suggested, they have been subjected to intense scrutiny—often more than their White counterparts faced. With more diversity in accreditation leadership in recent years, however, there has been an effort to bring about fairness.[30]

In 1992, President Goodman decided to leave the institution. He had enjoyed his time as the leader of the medical school, but he wanted to try something new. Returning to the plan he had made before accepting the presidency of Morehouse School of Medicine, Goodman moved to Seattle and acquired a Jiffy Lube franchise.

Nelson McGhee Fills a Gap

With Goodman leaving, the medical school had to quickly find a replacement. They looked to a man with outstanding connections to both the Black college and the medical community. Nelson McGhee, a 1951 graduate of historically Black Talladega College, was their choice. McGhee had earned his master's degree from Atlanta University in 1953, and he held an MD from Meharry Medical College and a PhD from Union Graduate School. Before serving as interim president of Morehouse School of Medicine, McGhee was the vice president of community affairs and a professor in the Department of Obstetrics and Gynecology. He had served as a member of the Board of Trustees, and he chaired the committee that oversaw the construction of a new building, Gloster Hall.

The Board of Trustees asked McGhee to serve as interim president until January 1993. During that time, he played a key role in securing federal matching funds for the medical school, and as a result it was able to expand its clinical programs. McGhee was also instrumental in advancing the institution's relationship with Grady Memorial Hospital and Emory's School of Medicine. After serving as president, McGhee returned to the faculty.[31]

According to Walter Sullivan, vice president of sponsored programs, McGhee was well liked by faculty and staff—"always jovial, he was cracking jokes, but not in a silly way."[32] Some thought that McGhee wanted to assume the presidency of the institution. In fact, Louis Sullivan remembers McGhee trying to convince him not to come back as president, saying that Sullivan was now "too big" for Morehouse School of Medicine and would have many opportunities at larger institutions, including corporations. Nevertheless, Sullivan was recruited back to the medical school by the chair of the Board of Trustees. Sullivan's heart was still involved in the continued development of Morehouse School of Medicine, and he saw this as an opportunity to finish what he started. Upon his return from Washington, on January 21, 1993, he took the reins of the institution once again.[33]

Louis Sullivan Resumes the Presidency

President Sullivan would continue leading Morehouse School of Medicine until 2002. Energized by his experience in Washington, Sullivan started to build the institution's endowment. Following up on Goodman's commitment to primary care, he secured a gift of $1.2 million from Trustee Sally

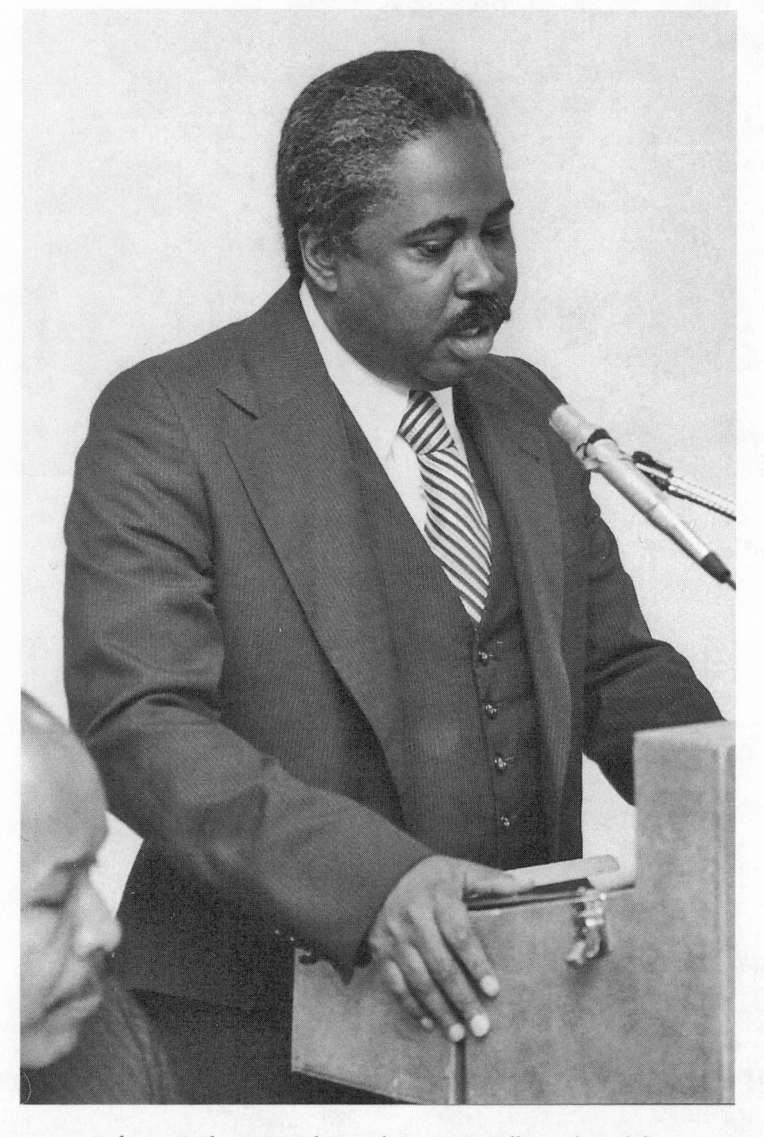

Nelson McGhee, MD, PhD, with Louis W. Sullivan (*lower left*).

Hambrecht and her husband, William, for the first endowed chair at More-house School of Medicine. He also established the George and Barbara Bush Chair in Neuroscience with a gift of $1.5 million from a Houston-based foun-dation; the donor had been a classmate of George H. W. Bush's at Yale.[34] And he raised $23 million to build the National Center for Primary Care, which was renamed the Louis W. Sullivan Center for Primary Care after his retire-

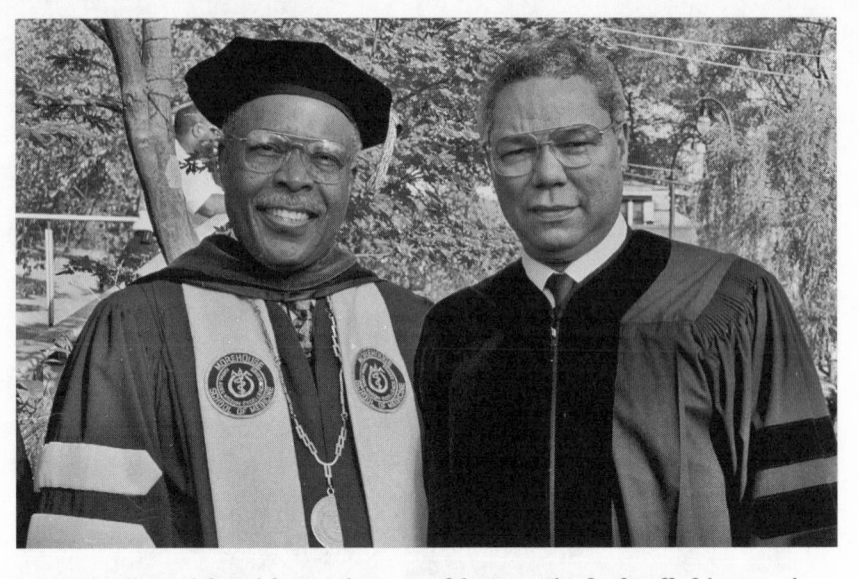

Louis W. Sullivan (*left*) and former chairman of the Joint Chiefs of Staff of the Armed Services, General Colin Powell (*right*), at the Morehouse School of Medicine commencement, 1994. Photograph courtesy of Horace C. Henry.

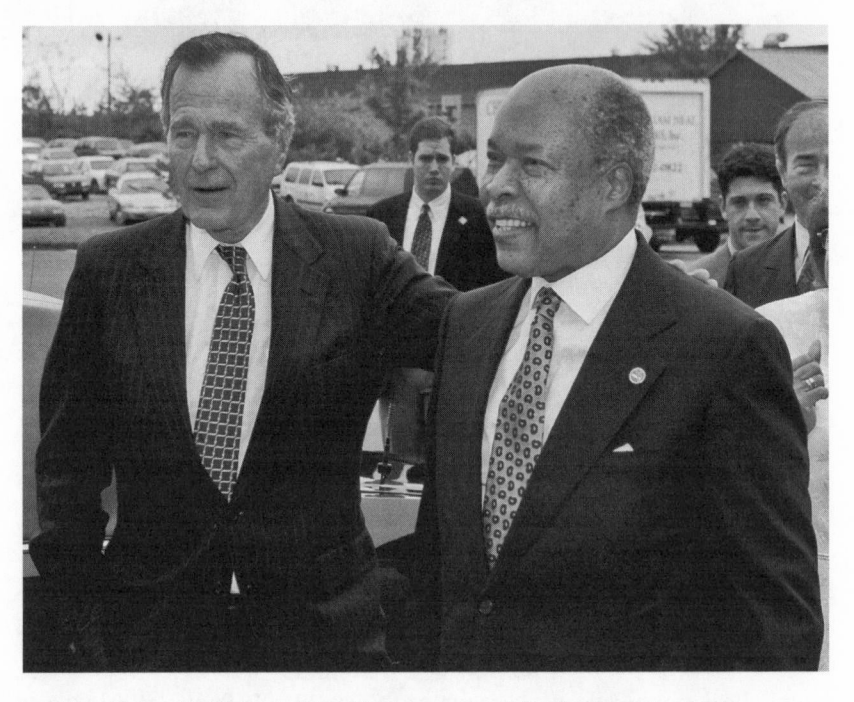

President George H. W. Bush (*left*) visits Morehouse School of Medicine for the groundbreaking ceremonies, National Center for Primary Care, 1999. Also pictured is Louis W. Sullivan (*right*). Photograph courtesy of Wilford Harewood.

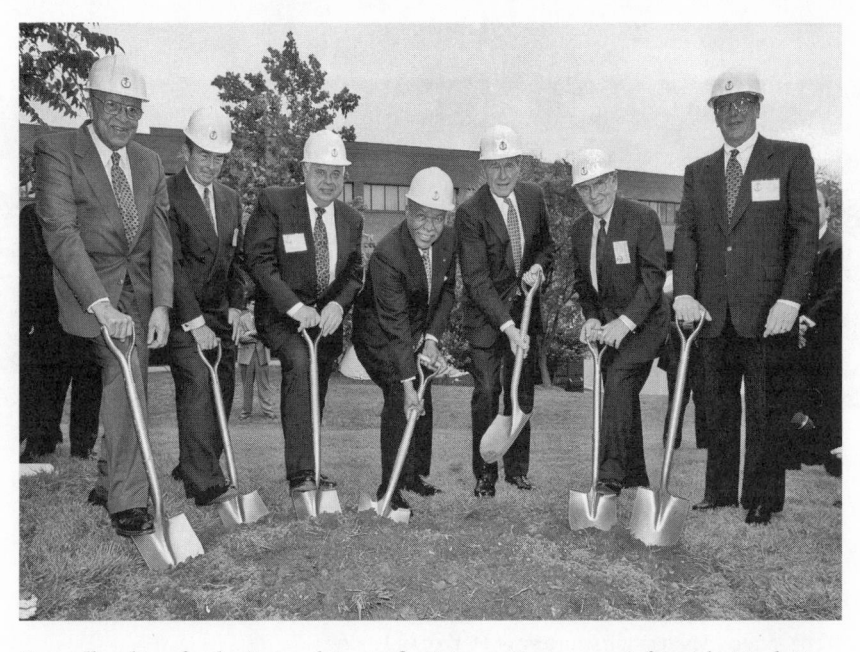

Groundbreaking for the National Center for Primary Care, 1999. *Left to right*, Hugh M. Gloster, president of Morehouse College; Charles Heimbold, CEO of Bristol Myers Squibb (vice-chairman of campaign); Desi De Simone, CEO of 3M Corporation (chairman of campaign); Louis Sullivan, president of Morehouse School of Medicine; President George H. W. Bush; Gerald Blakeley, chairman of the Morehouse School of Medicine Board of Trustees; Lew Polatt, CEO of Hewlett Packard (vice-chairman of campaign).

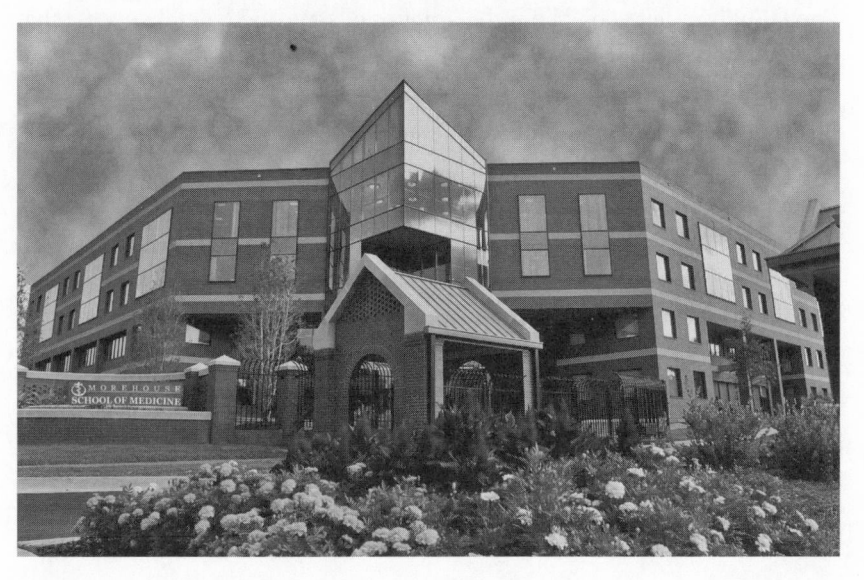

The Louis W. Sullivan National Center for Primary Care (dedicated September 1, 2002). Photograph courtesy of Horace C. Henry.

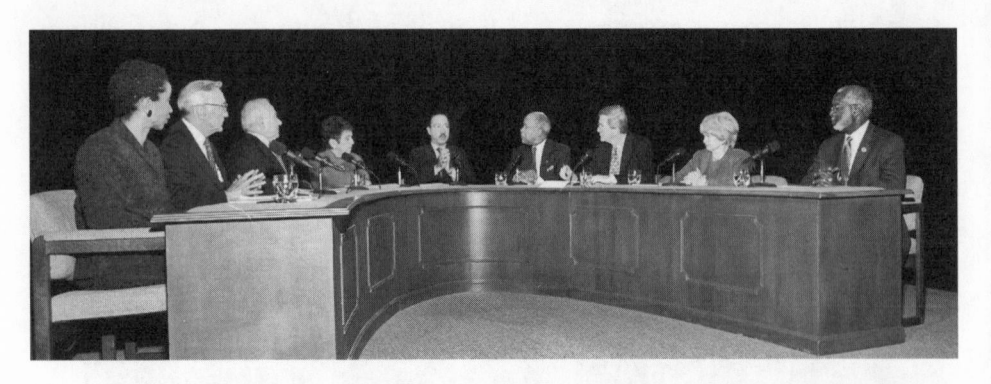

A conference of former U.S. Secretaries of Health and Human Services at Morehouse School of Medicine, April 2002. *Left to right,* Helene Gayle, President of CARE; Secretary Richard S. Schineiker (1981–1983); Secretary Joseph A. Califano Jr. (1977–1987); Secretary Donna E. Shalala (1993–2000); moderator George Strait; Secretary Louis W. Sullivan (1989–1993); Secretary David Mathews (1975–1977); Secretary Margaret M. Heckler (1983–1985); David Satcher, Surgeon General, U.S. Public Health Service (1993–2000). Photograph courtesy of Horace C. Henry.

ment in 2002.[35] According to his wife, Ginger: "he was always fundraising for these magnificent buildings at Morehouse School of Medicine. The Center for Primary Care was his prize. He completed that building and stepped down as president and brought in a new president."[36] By the time he left in 2002, Sullivan felt good about the amount of state and federal support that the medical school had received, but he knew the institution needed even more private support. In an effort to assist his successor, Sullivan created a Board of Visitors, made up of Atlanta business leaders, whose purpose was to recruit talent and raise funds in Atlanta.

From 1989 to 2002, Sullivan left, others stepped up, and Sullivan returned. But the medical school stayed a steady course, building relationships with alumni and the local community, recruiting a strong student body, adding buildings and research institutes, and expanding its fundraising capabilities.[37] It was clear that Morehouse School of Medicine had matured, and there was a sense in the institution as a whole of what its priorities should be. This institutional cohesion would be of great benefit during the turbulent years to come.

CHAPTER SIX

A Controversy Erupts

The man Morehouse's Board of Trustees chose to be Sullivan's successor had once aspired to be a Methodist minister, and he had the warm and friendly personality to match that aspiration. Hand picked by Sullivan himself, James Gavin stepped into the leadership role at Morehouse School of Medicine on July 1, 2002. A son of Alabama, he received his undergraduate education from historically Black Livingstone College in North Carolina. With encouragement from his mentors, he changed his career plans and became one of the first African Americans to enroll in Emory University's graduate programs. He earned a PhD in biochemistry from Emory in 1970 and an MD from Duke University in 1975.[1]

By the time he came to the Morehouse presidency, Gavin was a well-known endocrinologist, specializing in diabetes. He was also a senior scientific officer at the Howard Hughes Medical Institute. Sullivan, who "heavily recruited" Gavin as a candidate, did not know him well but had heard him speak and noted his excellent reputation.[2] At first Gavin was not interested in the position, but as he learned of the good work that Morehouse School of Medicine was doing, especially in mentoring and producing minority physicians, his interest grew. From Gavin's perspective, the medical school was very well networked in philanthropy, in big science, and in medicine.[3] He thought that he could put his own stamp on an institution that was already operating at a high level. For his part, Sullivan saw Gavin as someone with a background similar to his own—that of an academician. "Gavin was the ideal candidate," Sullivan said, "articulate, a great personality, terrific scholar, and engaging. I figured what he needed to know as an administrator, he could learn, like I did."[4]

James Gavin

Sullivan was enthusiastic about bringing someone of Gavin's stature to the medical school, but his excitement would soon wane.[5] The two men had very different perspectives on the institution and its leadership. Sullivan explained that he wanted what was best for the school and "expected Gavin to build on the legacy he had left in place."[6] Gavin, though, was not content to merely live in Sullivan's shadow. He said:

> I didn't really know the culture of the school of medicine and certainly didn't realize the extent to which everything about the school was essentially Lou Sullivan. It was his signature, it was his culture. And that is not a negative thing, it simply is what happens when you have a person who was the sort of big figure that Lou is, driving the development and the early growth of an institution. The medical school had evolved into a place where the board did more listening to him than he did to the board, which was not the kind of governance I was used to.[7]

Friends told Gavin that nothing he had done in the past would prepare him for the presidency of the Morehouse School of Medicine, but he decided not to heed their warning. He began the job in July 2002.[8] To prepare for his new role, Gavin made a few visits to the Atlanta campus. But Sullivan had wanted him to visit more often and become better oriented to Atlanta; Sullivan also wanted to mentor the new president. Gavin had never really lost contact with Atlanta and had regularly visited the city, since the Emory University Howard Hughes Medical Institute unit was under his supervision for a number of years. Believing that his time at Emory and subsequent interactions were enough to establish a connection to Atlanta, Gavin did not spend more time there.[9] "Lou wanted to be my patron of sorts and introduce me around," Gavin said, "and that just wasn't my style."[10] Gavin saw himself as quite different from Sullivan: "Whereas Lou had come up through government and appointed positions, I was a much more straightforward academic. I knew that there was very little likelihood that I would run anything in the same way that Lou did." The misconception these two men had of each other was stark. In fact, Sullivan had been an academic all his life until stepping into the medical school leadership position; he did not work in government until tapped by President Bush years after arriving at Morehouse.[11]

When Gavin arrived, Sullivan tried to get on the new president's calendar. He thought it was his role to orient Gavin, just as Morehouse College president Hugh Gloster had done for him. "Before I came to Morehouse," Sullivan said, "I had never been a president, and while I was a native Atlantan, I had never functioned or interacted with the business community. So my thought was that I would transfer the relationships that I had to him."[12] But at the end of the third meeting, Gavin said: "Lou, you and I operate differently. I like to try and figure out things myself and then, if I need help, then

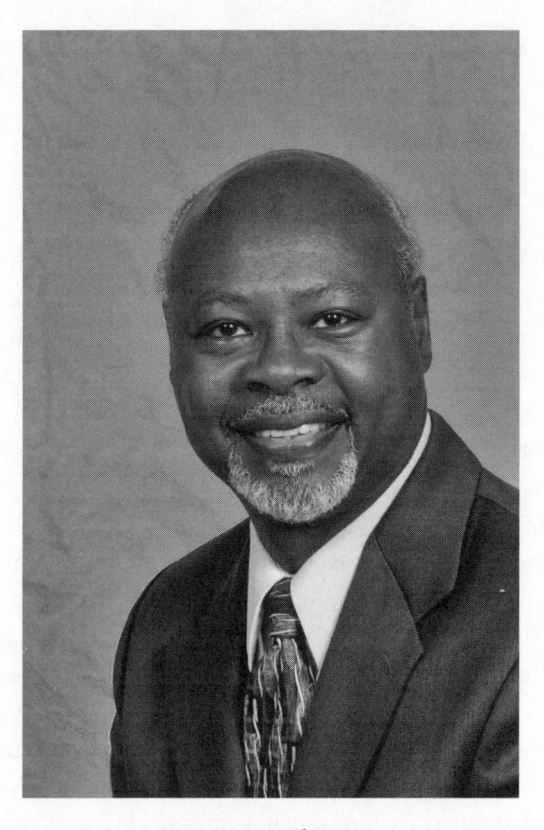

James Gavin, PhD, MD.

ask for it. So if you don't mind, let me just proceed, and if I need some help from you, I will call you."[13] This solidified a rift between the two strong leaders.

Sullivan might not have appreciated the difference between his role upon coming to Morehouse College and Gavin's role in coming to Morehouse School of Medicine. Whereas Sullivan came in as a program dean and was mentored by Hugh Gloster, the president of Morehouse College, Gavin came to the freestanding medical school as its president. Most college presidents do not appreciate a former president offering advice unless they seek it. On the other hand, deans typically join a college or university hoping to be "shown the ropes" by the president and others at the institution.[14]

As the new president, Gavin had to contend with a $4.5 million cut from its annual state grant. "When you're talking about a school with a total [unrestricted] operating budget of $60 million, that's a huge loss," Gavin said, "especially because the loss came during the middle of the fiscal year, when the money had already been budgeted for specific programs."[15] This difficulty convinced Gavin that the school relied too much on state and federal funds. Gavin said candidly, "We needed to increase the flow of revenue from the private sector, and in order for that to happen, the community has to own us."[16] Although considerable work had been done by the previous presidents to create relationships with local businesses and leaders, Gavin felt that there was still a rift. He talked with many people in the Atlanta community, and they left him with the impression that they did not understand the school. They knew its very strong national reputation, but Gavin felt they were not familiar enough with its local contributions. The medical school was still seen as aligned with Washington rather than with Atlanta.[17] Years had elapsed since James Goodman's widespread speaking engagements across the Atlanta community; moreover Sullivan, during his second administration, had raised more money from national foundations and the federal government than from local citizens. Gavin thought that more local ownership would lead to increased funding from Atlanta and Georgia foundations, whose paltry donations were, in his words, "shameful."[18] He set up a public relations effort specifically designed to change this situation. The program included appearances on television, radio, and in churches; it also opened up the campus for community involvement.[19] A lesson to be learned from the medical school's experience is that no matter how much its mission is rooted in the local community, an institution must make constant efforts to nurture its town-gown relationships. In fundraising, Gavin noted that "we added hundreds of names to the donor list of the school and boasted a mantra that we were "a small medical school with outrageous ambition," and it really caught on."[20]

According to members of the medical school staff, President Gavin was a "master of language," with a great sense of humor and the ability to connect with others.[21] Under Gavin's leadership the school convinced the W. K. Kellogg Foundation to base its Community Voices program at the institution. The $18 million program, which had branches at the University of North Carolina at Chapel Hill, the University of Iowa, UCLA, and Morehouse School of Medicine, was set up with the goal of moving the nation toward universal health care by 2008. Because of Morehouse School of Medicine's dedication to primary medical care, Kellogg thought the institution was highly qualified to host a program devoted to working at the community level to reach underserved populations.[22] Although Gavin had his critics, he was able to bring acclaim to the Atlanta medical school.

Gavin also sought money to expand the institution's PhD programs. He noticed that the medical school had a robust research program, but it was built on the shoulders of the principal investigators; there were no trainees and no postdoctoral students. Moreover, there were very few graduate students to assist with research.[23] According to Gavin:

> One of the things that I emphasized to the institute directors and the research center directors was that you can't build a sustainable program of excellence and research without a pipeline of trainees, and so we really focused on increasing the size and depth of the PhD program, increasing the attractiveness of the institution for graduate students.[24]

In an effort to strengthen the School of Medicine's programs and centers, Gavin undertook and supervised a comprehensive program review. He was anticipating reaccreditation and, as a result, he challenged every program, from maintenance to the dean's office, to justify its role and its contributions to the medical school.[25] These efforts helped faculty and staff find strengths and weaknesses across the institution.

Gavin's data-driven, team approach to leadership was well received by most of the staff. "I had a good relationship with the staff," he said, "because I dealt with them on a level playing field. And this is not because I campaigned as some kind of populist. I started out as a Methodist preacher, so fairness and issues of justice are very important to me."[26] Gavin saw himself as a crusader for reform at the medical school; he felt that people "on the lower rungs" of the staff had been treated unfairly in the past. When he tried to achieve salary parity among the lower- and high-level administrators, he felt "the wrath of more senior-level people." Gavin refused to give the senior administrators a raise until he was able to offer the day-to-day staff a pay increase. He said: "I would have thought the senior-level people would have cheered me as a hero. They wanted to put me on a stake and burn me." Any time a president attempts to make large-scale systemic change at an institution, he or she will feel backlash from those who benefit from the status quo.[27]

Despite, or, in Gavin's mind, because of his successes, a "hornet's nest of resentment" formed on the campus.[28] From Sullivan's perspective, Gavin's leadership was not satisfactory.[29] The crux of the matter was that the two leaders had a different way of leading and communicating. President Gavin felt that he was constantly under a microscope, since Sullivan was on the Board of Trustees and Executive Committee. Sullivan, Gavin said, "provided a sort of running critique of my performance." He added, "I don't want to sound like my presidency was a litany of sour grapes, but I think what it really represented was an institution where the governance structure was not ready for any new leadership."[30] Gavin and Sullivan had personalities that did not mix well; Gavin said, "Lou is the kind of person who doesn't accept no, and he is [as] tenacious as a person could ever be."[31] Because Sullivan was present on campus, he was a constant reminder of "what the president was supposed to do and be and act like every day."[32] The situation into which Gavin stepped was intensely difficult.[33]

In addition, Gavin was having trouble working with the Board of Trustees. He described it as an increasingly dysfunctional interaction. In the summer of 2004, Gerald Blakeley and Anthony Welters, the board chair and vice-chair, respectively, called Gavin to a meeting at Welters's office in New York City. They scheduled the meeting on a day when thousands of minority students were coming to the medical school for a recruitment event, and Gavin had planned to address them. The president told Blakeley and Welters that the day was not convenient for him, but they insisted that he fly to New York.[34]

During the meeting, Blakely informed Gavin that the board was not pleased with his performance as president. Gavin reported that Blakely focused on the inability to get along with Sullivan as a key reason for Gavin's lack of success. As Gavin recalls, Blakely thought the best way to move forward was for Gavin to resign. He refused and said he had no reason to do that. He reminded the two that he had not been given a performance evaluation despite asking for one, so the notion of inadequate performance was not established. The meeting ended with Gavin telling Blakely and Welters that he needed time to think about their conversation. According to Gavin, within a week he received a letter from Blakely that said: "Since you would not cooperate, since you're unwilling to adhere to the board's wishes, we will have to take steps to remove you from the position of president."[35] Infuriated by the letter, Gavin wrote a detailed reply, describing the meeting in New York that took place a week earlier, and sent it to Blakely, Welters, and his own attorney.

In the end, by mutual agreement, Gavin submitted his resignation in December 2004. According to Sullivan, "he definitely considers me the person responsible for his difficulties with the board, and I readily face up to that."[36] Gavin said:

> I really lost respect for Sullivan the more I got to know and understand the kind of
> person that he is, and that is not to diminish his rather substantial contributions.

He's done some remarkable things, but I think that there are times when you really
need to have the benefit of some distance from your heroes. You don't need to know
a whole lot more than their public persona.[37]

Upset with Gavin's termination, Clinton Warner resigned from the board.
He felt that Gavin was the right man to lead the medical school and should
have been given more time to settle in.[38] Warner also thought that Gavin and
board chair Blakely could have worked things out—that their disagreement
was not something that needed to be aired in a board meeting—and that the
difference between Sullivan and Gavin was a matter of style and personality,
not substance. Warner said:

[Gavin and Blakely] needed to go off and fight it out together. Not in the board room.
They needed to come to a conclusion that they both could support and then go back
to the board. Any differences could have been worked out. He just had a different
way of leading than folks were used to—it wasn't wrong.[39]

The leadership struggle at Morehouse School of Medicine surfaced in the
public arena, bringing unwanted publicity to the institution. On December
18, 2004, the *Atlanta Journal-Constitution* ran a front page story under the
headline "Morehouse Med School to Ax Chief," with James Gavin's picture
front and center.[40] According to the article, the medical school's Board of
Trustees had "taken steps to oust the school's popular president, a move supporters of the institution fear could threaten its accreditation."

The article further reported that, at a town hall meeting at the medical
school earlier that month, it was announced that Gavin would be replaced by
an interim president—former U.S. surgeon general David Satcher—"as soon
as a mutually agreeable resolution is reached between Gavin and the school."
Satcher was director of the National Center for Primary Care and had a history with the institution, having served as chair of the Department of Community Medicine from 1979 to 1982.

In the *Journal-Constitution* article, Gavin described himself as the victim
of a vendetta; he said that "there was 'no valid claim for a performance-based
complaint' against him and that board members 'simply want me gone.'"
The article stated that Gavin explained that he "had clashed with board members who launched a relentless campaign to damage [his] credibility and
erode [his] integrity. . . . He has been a target of professional slights and al-
legations without substance dating from his earliest days as president. Board
members have accused him of everything from being inaccessible to faculty

members to being a bad fund-raiser." It noted that Gavin had refused to re-sign and was forced out of his position.

In spite of a few loud voices against him, President Gavin, known for his friendly and warm disposition, had considerable support among the faculty and staff.[41] At the town hall meeting where Gavin's departure was announced, more than 300 people from the medical school and the surrounding com-munity gave him a standing ovation. According to David Satcher:

> There was a real uproar over Jim's situation, and we had this big meeting with a large audience. I had already decided that I would take the interim presidency, so the board was able to put me in between them and the staff. I explained to the staff that I didn't seek this role and I was not a disciple of Lou Sullivan or Jim Gavin. I was only concerned about the institution. Some people complained about this be-cause they thought they should have been given an opportunity to confront the board. Gavin was very popular, and they wanted to have at the board. He just had that kind of personality.[42]

The school was scheduled to undergo a review of its accreditation in Feb-ruary 2005, and a group of senior faculty members wrote a letter to the Board of Trustees on December 9, 2004, expressing grave concern about changing the institution's leadership at a "critical time in the review process."[43] They argued that "a decision to remove a sitting president in the midst of review for accreditation will have a damaging impact on our school. Such actions threaten the outcome of our impending accreditation visit."[44]

Gavin also had support beyond the medical school, and Atlanta community leaders came to the town hall meeting. They said that Gavin had been a positive force in the city, pointing specifically to his outreach work—something that Gavin is proud of when he reflects on his experience at the medical school.[45] Just before the town hall meeting, many of these community leaders sent a memo in support of Gavin to the Board of Trustees.[46]

People in the local community criticized the Board of Trustees and its treatment of Gavin, and some wanted to demonstrate and confront the board.[47] In addition to the community leaders at the town hall meeting, Gavin met with members of local churches, who understood what was going on and wanted to register their strong protest. Gavin recalled:

> For the first time in their memory, they felt like the school was really part of the community, and they were ready to take to the streets like old demonstrations of the civil rights era. And I said no, no way. I said that would simply spill the blood of this

institution all over the streets of Atlanta, and the *Atlanta Journal-Constitution* would sell 200,000 more copies, but the institution would be permanently scarred, and that's just not why I came here.[48]

Though he discouraged them from protesting, Gavin made it clear to the church leaders that, in his view, he had done nothing wrong.[49]

Many leaders, faced with this type of unfortunate situation, might have left the city as quickly as possible, but Gavin and his wife stayed. He said:

This community has been an extremely warm and supportive community. I'm blessed beyond measure in the sense that I'm able to do what I want to do, and am actually enjoying doing what I'm doing in ways that I have not been in years, and my relationship with Emory has always been strong. I'm on the Board of Trustees there, and I'm heading the graduate school component of the capital campaign.[50]

In retrospect, said David Satcher: "Gavin and Sullivan are both good people. It's just one of those situations. I think it's fair to say that Lou had difficulty transitioning out of the presidency." Satcher also noted that from the very beginning of Gavin's presidency, he had a rocky relationship with the Board of Trustees: "It was Lou Sullivan's board, so they gave Jim a rough time. I'm not saying Jim was blameless. I know Jim had trouble getting started."[51]

Beyond his slow start, President Gavin's major mistake may have been that he did not bring his own leadership team with him to the medical school. This is a common strategy for presidents, because it is essential that executives have a trusted group of people surrounding them and in their corner when they have to make tough decisions.[52] "You have to have your own team," Satcher said. "Even right up top—the people working with Gavin were people who worked with Lou for years. It was a difficult transition."[53]

The disputes between Gavin and Sullivan were complex, and they involved substantial differences in leadership styles and personalities. Sullivan wanted to stay involved with the institution he developed and shaped, while Gavin wanted to make his own mark and break free from the previous administration. The disagreements between them point to larger problems at founder-driven institutions. At times, having the founder present can keep new people from contributing in the ways they feel are best. In this case, Gavin's contributions to the medical school were not insignificant—he attracted new supporters and generated a community spirit. But he was not comfortable having the institution's previous leader involved in the school. It would take the next president to finally resolve the problem of Sullivan's continued participation.

CHAPTER SEVEN

Recovering from Turmoil

Upon James Gavin's dismissal from Morehouse School of Medicine, David Satcher was asked to serve as interim president. Satcher had a formidable reputation. From 1998 to 2001, during the Clinton administration, he served as the sixteenth Surgeon General of the United States; at the same time, he was Assistant Secretary of Health in the U.S. Department of Health and Human Services. Earlier, from 1993 to 1998, Satcher was director of the Centers for Disease Control and Prevention. Many at the medical school looked to Satcher because of his leadership experience at other medical schools: he was dean at Charles R. Drew Medical School for 2 years and president of Meharry Medical College for 12. Satcher was also a 1963 Morehouse College graduate, and he received his MD and PhD from Case Western Reserve University in 1970.

Satcher was a natural choice for interim president. He had a good relationship with both Sullivan and Gavin. He had written a letter of support for Gavin during the turmoil and served as a confidant to him: "Whenever he got in trouble with the board, he would call me because he needed somebody to vent with."[1] On the other hand, Satcher was close with Sullivan, who had been his mentor for years.

Having led Meharry Medical College, Satcher was not keen to serve as the Morehouse School of Medicine president. In fact, it was the last thing he wanted to do. Satcher said, however:

> The faculty members told me if I did not step up and become interim president, they were going to leave because people were very concerned. They were concerned about Lou. They were concerned about the board. And they felt like Lou and the board had been very unfair to Jim Gavin, and to a certain extent I agreed that he had not been given a chance to be successful.[2]

It was a combination of his love for the medical school and his respect for Sullivan that led Satcher to step into the presidency. He knew how hard Sullivan had worked to build the institution, and he did not want to stand by and see it erode.

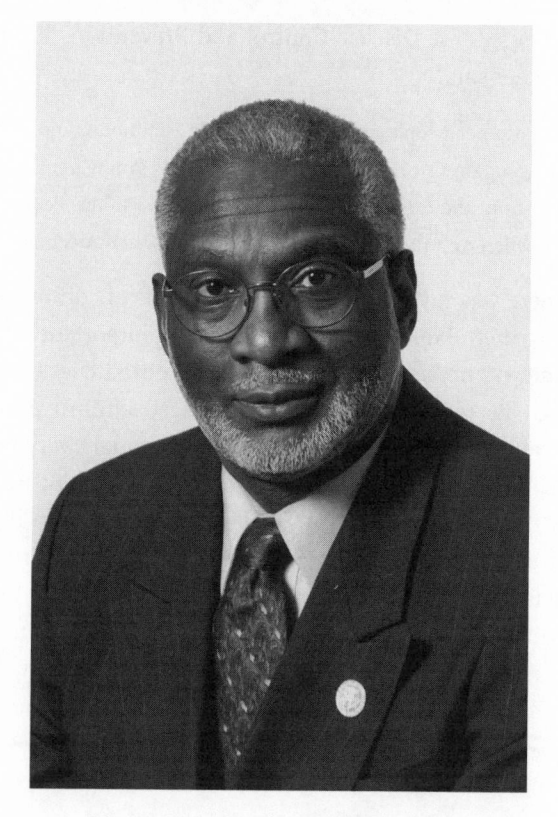

David Satcher, MD, PhD.

David Satcher

Satcher came to the presidency with more leadership experience than any of his predecessors, and he had a seasoned approach to leadership—he didn't have to learn on the job. In Satcher's words: "One of the first things that I do when I become a leader is figure out how I am going to put a team together. The longer you lead, the broader that team becomes."[3] To promote unity, Satcher brought the executive leadership together for monthly retreats, noting that "many of them didn't even know each other; they had never met each other in a team format—they had been operating in their individual silos."[4] Satcher wanted the institution to have a cohesive leadership structure so that it would be prepared for presidential leadership challenges in the future.[5] He developed this approach as president of Meharry Medical College and as director of the Centers for Disease Control and Prevention. "Every place that I've been," Satcher said,

> I have pulled together people to say, "This is your institution, and I want you to know what is going on." At Meharry, we had a monthly family hour that was open to everybody—from the executive vice president to the janitor. People knew that once a month when we had the family hours—that was their meeting.[6]

For Satcher there was no question about his means of communicating with staff and letting them know that they each had an important role to play.

Although he was president for only a short time, Satcher helped steer the school through its reaccreditation and increased alumni participation in the school's events.[7] And he also had to do some tough, very political work while interim president. Once Satcher took control, the Board of Trustees made it clear that they wanted Louis Sullivan to retire from his leadership role. Otherwise, the board thought, it would be difficult to recruit the kind of president the institution needed, because no one would want to take the job if they thought they would be subject to the same kind of treatment that Gavin had received. According to Satcher, "all over the country, the story was that Jim Gavin was a good man, well trained, and yet he couldn't succeed here, so why would other people want to come?"[8] The chair of the Board of Trustees, Anthony Walters, went to Satcher and asked him to ease Sullivan off the board.

Given that Satcher and Sullivan had been friends for quite a long time, the new interim president thought he could handle the situation easily:

> The first thing I did was sit down with Lou and talk and talk and talk about why I thought it was a really good idea for him to leave the board. But he never would agree to that. It came down to the trustees having to take a vote in the board meeting, and someone stood up and said, "Lou, why don't you spare us. We don't want to vote you off the board." So in the final analysis, he resigned.[9]

Satcher believes that Sullivan partly blames him for the forced resignation: "He probably feels that they couldn't have pulled that off without me. He probably thinks that it was my leadership that gave them the comfort to do that and gave them the credibility. And there's some truth to that, and I know that."[10] According to John Maupin, the medical school's president after Satcher: "David was really upfront with me. He said, 'I did this. I'm willing to admit it, and this is why Lou is mad at me.'"[11]

Although there are hard feelings between Satcher and Sullivan—both of whom brought immense acclaim to Morehouse School of Medicine—they also acknowledge one another's contributions. Satcher said: "There are very few people in the world I respect more than Lou. It pains me, really, that this happened."[12] In an effort to repair his once solid relationship with Sullivan, President Satcher proposed to the Board of Trustees that a building be named after the former leader—the National Center for Primary Care. Awkwardly, Satcher told Sullivan of the honor during the same meeting in which he asked him to leave the board. Reflecting on the situation, Satcher agrees that this wasn't the wisest strategy. He confesses: "It was in the same meeting, and I may have been playing little games with myself, trying to balance the message as number one, I think it's time for you to leave the board; number two, I think it's time that we really honor you."[13]

Angela Franklin, who served as dean of students under Sullivan, said: "The medical school was Lou's baby. He loves the school in a way that no other person ever loved that institution. I know it hurt him probably to see the chaos and confusion that happened as he stepped down, and my heart ached for him as that was happening." In Franklin's opinion, Sullivan was "pushed aside in a way that was not necessary and not called for." To this day, she has mixed feelings about those who were involved; she is adamant in her belief that the medical school would not exist if not for Louis Sullivan and saddened by how the controversy hurt the institution.[14]

After taking care of the situation with Sullivan, Satcher worked to prepare the institution for the reaccreditation process, which came two months after Gavin's dismissal. He began a series of meetings with students, faculty, and staff designed to boost cohesion on campus. He hosted community forums and brought Atlanta leaders to the school.[15] These meetings helped maintain the support that Gavin had garnered during his tenure, especially in the Black community.[16] Satcher was very diplomatic about working with different factions:

> I would begin every one of the community meetings by saying, "I know that some of you are supporters of Dr. Sullivan and some of you are supporters of Jim Gavin. I appreciate that. My concern is the institution, so what I want you to do is help me get this institution on track to survive the accreditation site visits." That was my attitude.[17]

On campus, Satcher made it clear to the students that their support was a vote of confidence in neither Louis Sullivan nor James Gavin, but in the institution as a whole. And the efforts to build unity worked. When the accreditation site visitors came, they said that they had never seen a group of students, staff, and faculty as enthusiastic about their institution. Morehouse School of Medicine received the maximum accreditation span of eight years.[18]

Satcher also worked to strengthen the alumni base, hoping to offset the institution's heavy reliance on federal and corporate funds.[19] He understood that more alumni giving would not only add to the bottom line but would be noticed and appreciated by corporations and foundations when deciding which institutions would receive funds from them.[20] When Satcher took office, however, only 8 percent of the alumni were giving to the medical school. "I made it very clear to them," Satcher said, that "the issue here is 'I need your name on the list.' I need you to say that you support this institution." He told the alumni that the size of the gift was not as important as the participation rate. The effort paid off: during Satcher's time as president, alumni giving quadrupled.[21] The consensus among faculty and staff was that interim president Satcher did a tremendous job at a critical time in the school's history. Board member Delutha King said:

> Dr. Satcher did what I thought was a remarkable job under the circumstances, coming in at a time when there was an attitude and environment that was not the greatest. He brought people together and moved the school forward in a very positive direction. The morale of the faculty and the student body seemed to improve greatly under his leadership.[22]

Choosing a New President

When the time came to choose the new president of the medical school, Sullivan said, interim president Satcher lobbied hard for the role. In fact, search committee chair Christopher Edwards urged him to submit his name for consideration. However, Sullivan said, Satcher did not want to submit his own name but preferred to be nominated, most likely because he did not want to risk the embarrassment of not getting the position.[23] In the end, the Board of Trustees chose John E. Maupin Jr. to be the fifth president of Morehouse School of Medicine. Maupin—who still leads the school at this writing—had over 30 years of experience in health care administration, public health, and academic medicine. He came to the institution with ample experience leading a medical school, having served as the president of Meharry Medical College for 12 years. He was the first Meharry alumnus and the second dentist to lead the Nashville institution.[24]

John Maupin

Maupin was no stranger to Morehouse, having served as the school's executive vice president and chief operating officer from 1989 to 1994—a position for which Louis Sullivan had recruited him.[25] In 1988, Maupin had been working at the Southside Community Health Center in Atlanta for roughly a year when board member Clinton Warner pulled him aside during a Georgia State Medical Association meeting. Warner said to him: "Lou Sullivan's going to give you a call. Don't ask any more questions. You've been prepared."[26] Maupin said: "Warner then walked away. It was like the Godfather pulled me aside and said I need to think about changing my career."[27] When Sullivan asked if he would serve as executive vice president, Maupin replied: "I'm flattered, but I just started at Southside Community Health Center, and my career goal was to lead a large, federally qualified health center such as Southside. Also, you know I've never worked in academia except as an adjunct faculty member. I have never wanted to pursue a career in academic medicine."[28] As Maupin recalls, President Sullivan said, in all seriousness:

> I'm not asking you to be dean; I'm asking you to run the administration and the support services of the school, and that's what your career has been about. Because you have a health background and you've worked with community health centers, you understand what we do. I want you to use your MBA, not your dental degree.[29]

After giving it some thought and consulting with his mentors—and after multiple attempts to convince Sullivan that he was not the right person for the job—Maupin decided to take the position.

Then Maupin learned that George H. W. Bush was considering Sullivan for the position of Secretary of Health and Human Services. Maupin was not pleased that the man who hired him was on his way to Washington, D.C., but he took the job anyway. On his first day of work, Maupin encountered a peculiar situation. James Goodman, who was to be president after Sullivan left, was frustrated with the medical school board. Goodman had refused the board's offer to make him interim president, stating that he would only lead the institution as president. Because Goodman refused to move into the president's office, Maupin could not get into his own office. He spent the first week sitting at a staff desk in the hallway, trying to schedule appointments with other members of the executive staff and faculty leadership to better understand their expectations of his role.[30] Recalling the tenor during his first stint as a Morehouse administrator, Maupin said: "In the five years I was

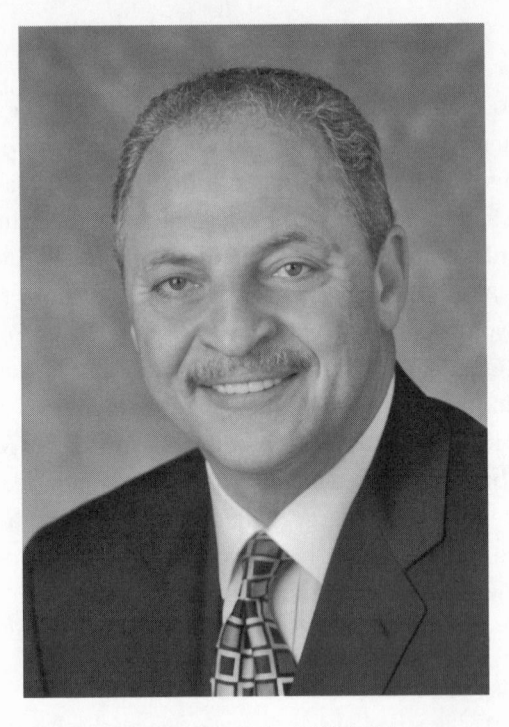

John E. Maupin Jr., DDS, MBA.

there, if you count Lou only once, not twice, there were three presidents, three deans, and three chief financial officers. So it was a period of rapid changing, a very disruptive leadership period, but also a great period of growth."[31] Many young institutions might not have survived the turmoil that Morehouse School of Medicine endured.[32] Maupin stayed on as executive vice president until 1994, and then moved on to the presidency of his alma mater, Meharry Medical School.

After serving his alma mater for more than a decade, Maupin was tapped by the Morehouse board in 2005. He had just finished a major capital campaign at Meharry and was ready to try new things when the inquiry came from the Board of Trustees. The representative of the search firm the board had hired made a high-pressure sales pitch: "What we hear is that you wouldn't have been able to be president of Meharry if it hadn't been for Morehouse. And if Morehouse thinks that you are appropriate for this time in its history, then you need to think about it. Don't you think you owe Morehouse, just like you owed your alma mater Meharry?"[33] Board members applied even greater pressure. One called Maupin and argued: "The issue between

Dr. Sullivan and Dr. Gavin was very disruptive to the institution. You are the only person who can bridge all the gaps. You know Gavin, you know Satcher, you know Sullivan. People know you from the past. You know the politics of Atlanta, you know the people of Atlanta."[34] The board members did not want someone who needed time to learn the ropes; they wanted a seasoned president.[35] And they wanted someone who had a good feel for the issues faced by predominantly and historically Black and community-oriented medical schools.[36]

After many conversations with his family, Maupin decided to take the position. Tragically, only a month after he did so, his son was killed in an auto accident. This incident led to a traumatic start for the new president and a period in his career that he describes as a roller coaster. "There's that saying about the most traumatic things in life being the death of a child, a new job, buying a home, and divorce," Maupin said. "Well, thank God that my wife didn't divorce me."[37] Compounding Maupin's anxiety in the first few months was the fact that the academic dean for the medical school would not be someone whom he hired. David Satcher, as interim president, had selected Eve J. Higginbotham for the position. President Maupin and Dean Higginbotham managed to get along, but they had to get used to each other's styles. As Maupin put it, "We had to come to an understanding of my perspective on her role in comparison to David Satcher's perspective."[38] Higginbotham left in 2010.

Maupin also had to cope with the rift that lingered between Louis Sullivan and David Satcher. "It was a very, very, very big divide," Maupin said, and he had to learn to manage it.[39] Although Sullivan was no longer on the Board of Trustees, he maintained an office in Atlanta and was still influential in Morehouse's affairs. There was also the residual impact of James Gavin's presidency. Although Satcher had worked to alleviate some of the tensions on campus and to bring people together, there were doubts about how Maupin would handle the divide between supporters of the former leaders.[40]

Maupin skillfully engaged all of the school's past leaders to move toward consensus. He said: "I told each of them, 'Your relationship with me has nothing to do with your relationship with each other.' I had to embrace these men respectfully but could not let them be in a position in which they would have undue influence on me."[41] Maupin decided to enlist Sullivan's aid by asking the former president to meet monthly for breakfast and to help him with people in the philanthropic world as well as federal officials.[42] He talked with Satcher about how the institution could best approach fundraising, given that both Maupin and Satcher would be looking for financial support in the community. (Maupin, of course, would be raising money for Morehouse, and Satcher would be garnering funds for the Satcher Health Leadership Institute.) They had to work closely to make sure they were not going to the same people for differing purposes. Maupin also had to convince Sullivan and Satcher to bury the hatchet sometimes, telling them that "from time to time you're both going to be on the same stage with me, because you're both past presidents."[43] For the most part, Maupin exacted a level of civility between the leaders. He noted that "both of them participated in my inauguration, and both of them are always recognized, and both of them are always invited."

Through all of the leadership changes and difficult transitions, the institution prevailed. But it had to weather rocky times. Morehouse School of Medicine faced many obstacles, including fundraising, expansion of its research facilities, and the need to enhance patient care at its affiliated facilities. Having unstable leadership made the regular functions of the institution more difficult. According to Maupin, "I quickly began to understand why the board wanted someone who understood the institution and the dynamics of the individuals involved with [it]."[44]

Despite having worked at the medical school before, Maupin took his time getting reacquainted with the institution—a strategy used by many successful presidents.[45] He sought to build the institution's technology, its research program, and its fundraising capacity. According to Mary Kay Murphy, the associate vice president for institutional advancement, "we're in a tremendous position to move forward on a capital campaign, but Dr. Maupin is insistent that we put the right things in place—a strategic plan, for example—before moving forward."[46] She added: "Maupin has given meticulous care and leadership to the strategic plan and fundraising strategies. He has created a board that can help him lead in the area of fundraising."[47] From her perspective, Maupin understood the basic tenets of board development: give, get, or get out of the way.[48] He spent considerable time interviewing potential board members and making sure that they understood their responsibility for fundraising. Maupin came to the institution at a time of turmoil. Under his leadership, the school has slowly come together, and the beginnings of consensus are evident.

Satcher and Maupin practiced sound leadership principles in their presidential roles. Satcher was able to mediate the situation between Sullivan and Gavin. He made a few regrettable decisions, but by and large, he was able to steer the institution through a crisis. And Maupin was able to quell conflict between the institution's two medical giants—Satcher and Sullivan—in order to move the medical school forward. Satcher turned the institution's attention toward its alumni and increasing their giving; Maupin focused on planning the growth of Morehouse School of Medicine.

CHAPTER EIGHT

Nurturing Students

Students who choose to attend Morehouse School of Medicine have typically been dedicated to primary care. They are committed to practicing medicine in communities that other people avoid. According to Walter Sullivan, Morehouse students "see a need to go into communities to keep people from taking buses and going halfway across town to see a physician."[1] Marjorie Smith, a longtime Morehouse faculty member and a member of the admissions committee, also described the Morehouse student as someone who understands the mission of the school and the importance of volunteering. Above all else, the institution looks to enroll students who want to give back to the community. This is not the norm at medical schools.[2] According to Dan Blumenthal, chair of the Community Health and Preventive Medicine Department, every medical school has far more applicants than it has slots. He said:

> If the admissions committee says the only things that are important are the MCAT [Medical College Admissions Text] and undergraduate grades—and some years they have—we end up with a different kind of student. But if they say MCAT scores and grades are important, but we also need to look at the personal essay that the student writes, we need to do an interview, and we need to know if the student believes in the mission of the school, then we end up with the best students for our institution.[3]

Blumenthal allowed that some students, after being admitted, are sidetracked by specialists who say, "You're too smart to go into family medicine," or by doctors who drive expensive cars and live in fancy houses. In Blumenthal's mind, however, Morehouse does "much better than most medical schools at finding idealistic students and helping them retain that idealism throughout medical school."[4] His claims are supported by research on socially responsible medical schools. According to a recent report in the *Annals of Internal Medicine*, for instance, minority physicians "provide relatively more care to minority and underserved populations compared with non-minority physicians." Those who graduate from historically Black medical schools are even more likely to reach out to underserved communities.[5]

Another reason that students choose Morehouse School of Medicine over

other institutions is the "family atmosphere and the friendliness and helpful-
ness of the administration and faculty."[6] Students feel empowered and mentored, and they believe faculty and staff want them to succeed. They don't get
the sense that they are being "weeded out," which is typical in medical schools
and science programs in general.[7] In this way, the atmosphere at Morehouse
School of Medicine is similar to that of other historically Black colleges and
universities.[8]

Lonnie Boaz, a member of the second class to be admitted, in 1979, and
former president of the alumni association, said: "I had a wonderful experience. The classes were small. We only had 24 students in our class. They
were in one building. There was a lot of interaction and communication between the two classes. The second-year class was extremely helpful to the
first-year class."[9] Even in 2010, class sizes were still small. According to Marjorie Smith, who began her career as a Morehouse faculty member in the
Pathology Department in 1978, the intentionally limited size of the classes,
and of the school overall, helped it to stay true to its mission. She hoped "that
it will stay relatively small—the students always comment that they hope we
never end up with classes of 150 students, like some other schools."[10]

Doug Paulsen, a member of the anatomy faculty, enjoyed getting to know
all of the students personally. He was able to see the students' strengths and
weaknesses early in their education. In fact, the atmosphere at Morehouse
was one of the reasons he has remained at the institution for a long period of
time.[11] Paulson is typical of the faculty in his approach to students. Even with
the entering class now hovering at 50 students, Paulson and others have an
open-door policy: "They just come into my office and plop themselves down
in the chair." He said he gives them advice not only on academic matters, but
on problems in their personal lives.[12]

A hallmark of Black colleges and universities is the nurturing effect these
institutions have on their students. Alumni cherish these experiences and
draw strength from them years after graduation.[13] Wayne Riley, an alumnus
of the School of Medicine (class of '93) and president of Meharry Medical
College, described his time at Morehouse thus:

> Medical school is a brutal process. It's not for the faint of heart. But there was some-
> thing different that happened at our institution. If you didn't go to class, people
> would notice, and they would call you and say, 'Everything okay?' That generally
> doesn't happen at other institutions. I don't know if you'd call it family atmosphere
> or a collective or a sense of shared victory, [but] that was special, and I don't think

other students at other institutions enjoyed the benefit of these types of educational experiences.[14]

Many Morehouse School of Medicine faculty members point to the caring nature of the professors as a reason for the institution's success: "Faculty who were willing to go that extra mile to find out where the student is and bring them to where they need to be. It's not lowering the bar for the students. It is doing what it takes to get them from where they are to where the bar is."[15] Not only did the institution nurture the students, it lit a fire in their bellies. Morehouse constantly reminded its students that there is a paucity of Black physicians in all specialties and that there was a scarcity of Black doctors developing public policy around health care. Physicians who graduated from Morehouse were expected to become leaders in their communities.[16]

In the first few years of the medical program, students benefited from close contact and relationships with Dean (and later President) Sullivan, who was highly visible on campus and within the day-to-day operations of the program. He and his wife, Ginger, hosted many picnics and parties at their home for students, including an annual welcome picnic and swim. Angela Franklin, who was dean of students during Sullivan's presidency, recalled: "We put it into the orientation schedule—pool party at the president's house. What is most amazing is that you would think that the president would just kind of stand around and watch the students swim. Sullivan, however, would step out with his flip-flops and his swimming shorts with his towel wrapped around his neck, and he would come out and host and welcome everyone to his home dressed like that." She added:

> I remember the first year, I put on my swimsuit with a wrap and thought, "OK, I'll be covered. I won't swim." But when he came out that first time dressed in his flip-flops—just regular department store flip-flops, not sandals, just flip-flops—he pranced around and was the first to dive in. The students were all taken aback, and then they all jumped in. He just loved every minute of it. It became the thing to look forward to every year.[17]

Sullivan looked forward to the students' lingering at his house and would invite them to play cards. According to those who knew him well, "it was the most unexpected response from a person like Lou Sullivan."[18] Lonnie Boaz, who attended the pool parties, said: "With Dr. Sullivan, we had a lot of interaction with him, and that was unusual. I had more interaction with Dr. Sullivan than I had with any of my high school principals, any dean or president of Vanderbilt. Dr. Sullivan was more than a dean or president; he was a friend to us."[19]

The pool party became a bit of a sore spot between Sullivan and James Gavin. During the first year of his presidency, Gavin did not have a house with a pool. According to Angela Franklin, Sullivan insisted on having the pool party anyway and volunteered his home. "It is tradition," he said. "We must have the pool party." Mirroring the other slights to Gavin's leadership, the president's pool party was hosted at the former president's house. Franklin said:

> Lou swam and Gavin did not. It was an awkward time that first year. Lou didn't really think anything of hosting the party at his house. He liked the way the students enjoyed the gathering each year. But you could imagine how this played out in Gavin's mind—"He still thinks he's president."[20]

Pool parties no longer take place at the Morehouse School of Medicine president's house, and some former students and staff think the culture of the school has lost something.[21]

As with any institution of higher education, faculty and student relationships are quite meaningful. Many of the former students of the medical school fondly remember their interactions with Marjorie Smith, the chair of pathology.[22] According to Lonnie Boaz: "People love her. I think the main thing was just her caring attitude, and that she really wanted the students to succeed, and the extra time that she put in with the students to make sure they really understood the material."[23] Wayne Riley concurred: "Marjorie Smith is a reflection of the commitment of faculty who came to Morehouse from other places and really believe in the mission of the institution—that the institution can have a broad impact in American higher education, and in academic medicine, and in community service, and they bought into that vision, as articulated by Dr. Sullivan."[24] He added: "Overall, the faculty embraced the mission with gusto. They nurtured us. They loved us. They criticized us. They kicked us in the butt. They did whatever they had to, to get us to the point where we crossed that stage at graduation and went out and hopefully changed the world."[25] Smith's approach—and that of the other teachers at Morehouse—was, she said, to get to know the students well: their faces and their names. Faculty members kept track of who was in their lectures and laboratories and who was not, following up with students who missed class. They communicated their high expectations to the students. In Marjorie

Smith's words, the faculty "don't pull any punches about what [the students] need to do and don't mollycoddle them."[26]

However, the medical school professors were more than just nice to the students, they were accessible to them—inside and outside the classroom. Boaz said:

> I don't think I had any one professor there that just came in and gave a lecture and walked out and left like he was through for the day. They were willing to stay after class to answer questions. We even had study sessions with professors, weekend study sessions, and that was the overall attitude—that they were there for us to make sure that we got the information, that we understood the information, and that we did well.[27]

Boaz compared his experience at Morehouse School of Medicine favorably with his undergraduate education at Vanderbilt University in Nashville, Tennessee:

> At Vanderbilt, particularly if you were premed, general chemistry and organic chemistry were large lecture classes where there were probably 200 to 300 students in each class. The professors would come in, give their lectures, and then walk out. Many times, that was the last time you saw them until the next class. There were very few study sessions. The situation was, "We present the information, and it is up to you to get it." Also, the competition between the premed students was pretty great. Basically, there wasn't a lot of camaraderie in terms of helping each other out.[28]

Boaz's experience at Vanderbilt is the typical medical school experience—large classes, little faculty-student interaction, and an intense sense of competition among the students.[29]

Boaz credits the pre-enrollment summer program at Morehouse School of Medicine with establishing the institution's family atmosphere. During this summer program, students took organic chemistry, general chemistry, and medical terminology. The summer program helped them get acclimated to sitting in class eight hours per day. According to Boaz: "That summer program was taught by Ray Barreras, who was one of the first instructors we met when we got there. It was his personality and attitude that let us know we were there as a family, and we would work to try to get everyone through rather than competing against one another."[30]

Boaz and other alumni found the atmosphere at Morehouse conducive to a great medical education experience:

> All of my memories of Morehouse are positive. I would have to say that definitely my two years were the best two years of education I ever had. I think it's the atmo-

sphere there. Normally, your first two years of medical school should be your hardest two years of school. But not at Morehouse. I enjoyed the atmosphere, my classmates, and everything about the place.[31]

According to Walter Sullivan, Louis Sullivan's brother and Morehouse's vice president of sponsored programs, the school was characterized by personal attention to students as well as "tremendous buy-in by faculty and administrators."[32] The institution's small size allows professors to monitor individual growth among students, and this gives both groups a sense of pride and accomplishment.[33]

The ability to shower students with personalized attention is the result not only of Morehouse School of Medicine's small size, but also of the tradition of challenge and uplift that has characterized its parent institution for over a century. Morehouse School of Medicine was an offshoot of Morehouse College, an institution with a rich tradition of graduating successful men—many of whom became leaders of the medical school. It is no surprise that Morehouse School of Medicine developed a similarly nurturing environment. The "Morehouse Mystique" spilled over to the medical school, providing an academically challenging and socially supportive educational environment for young people who wanted to pursue a career in medicine.

Conclusion

Morehouse School of Medicine was built in the spirit of all of those pioneers in African American medicine who lived decades earlier—Black students who braved the often hostile climate at historically White colleges and universities, and African American doctors who, against the odds, established their own medical schools and private practices in rural communities throughout the United States. Unlike its predecessors, however, Morehouse School of Medicine was formed during a time of increased racial cooperation and growing respect for African American intellect and contributions. President Gloster of Morehouse College was convinced that such an institution was needed and would thrive. Unlike his counterpart, Thomas Jarrett at Atlanta University, Gloster believed in the spirit of the medical school idea and was willing to take a risk, based on his institution's reputation and its track record, in the production of future medical students.

The Morehouse medical school idea represents an ideal convergence of time and place. Morehouse College itself was a focal point of the Black intelligentsia, graduating prominent leaders and thinkers, including Martin Luther King Jr.; as such, it offered an excellent location for the new institution. The College boasted many graduates who were physicians—some of whom occupied important positions in research and government. These alumni also provided a leadership base on which the new medical school could be founded. It is interesting to consider that even after separating from Morehouse College, the medical school retained the Morehouse brand name, knowing that it would lend prestige and instant recognition to the institution.

The Morehouse medical school idea came to fruition at a time of transition between segregation and integration. The path of the nation was uncertain. The extreme racial hostilities exemplified by Strom Thurmond, George Wallace, and, in Georgia, Lester Maddox were giving way to a more pragmatic approach to race relations. Yet the racial animus that stood behind the Blacks' lack of access to medicine and medical education remained. White medical schools were still not admitting Blacks in numbers significant enough to stem the inequalities in the field, and in 1970 there were still 13,810 Black people for every Black doctor in Georgia. It was clear that if African Americans were to close these gaps in medical care, they would have to take matters into their own hands.

In the three decades since it admitted its first class, Morehouse School of Medicine has had a significant impact on American medical education and on the delivery of medical care. First and foremost, the institution is dedicated to primary care, especially in rural and urban underserved areas. Each year it sends students into the field who are committed to providing services to those who may not be able to afford them. According to former ambassador Andrew Young: "The Morehouse School of Medicine model is basically that you are there primarily to serve people who don't have much money. Morehouse teaches family medicine at its best."[1] As shown by the school's records and confirmed by the American Medical Association, among all medical schools, Morehouse has the highest percentage of graduates going into primary care—between 65 and 70 percent annually—demonstrating that it is true to its mission.[2]

Another of Morehouse School of Medicine's contributions is the production of doctors who are African Americans or members of other minority groups. A small number of medical schools in the United States are responsible for graduating the majority of Black doctors, and Morehouse stands prominently among these institutions.[3] New doctors of color are vital to the health of Black communities across the nation and, in Morehouse's case, across the state of Georgia and throughout the South. Former Georgia governor Joe Frank Harris said: "The medical school has had a very positive impact on the state due to all of the physicians they have educated over the years. Many of them have stayed here in the state of Georgia, and many have addressed a lot of the underserved in rural areas and, of course, the underserved right here in the city of Atlanta."[4]

Because the medical school sprang from historically Black Morehouse College, it retained the unique advantages offered by this type of institution. Beginning in the 1980s, researchers identified characteristics of Black colleges that help students to succeed. These include a challenging yet supportive environment and a faculty that nurtures its students. The schools are also known for meeting students at whatever level they are academically and helping them to reach the bar of standards necessary to do well in their courses. Black institutions have enrolled students who might not otherwise be admitted to college, yet these same students, upon graduation, have been more likely to pursue graduate and professional degrees.[5] Most importantly, African American students who enroll in Black colleges come to study at places where their own culture and background is at the center of the learning experience. Rather than being cast adrift in an unfamiliar environment, most Black college students feel empowered, knowing that they are walking in the footsteps of previous generations of Black scholars and intellectuals.[6]

Using the knowledge they have gained and modeling their teachers' sense of responsibility and care, graduates of Morehouse School of Medicine are contributing to society's need for culturally competent doctors. According to the 2004 Sullivan Commission report, which focused on minorities in the health care professions: "In today's modern health care facilities, people from diverse cultures and social experiences cross paths. Understanding the unique and indispensable role that minority health providers play in health care delivery requires a fundamental appreciation of the powerful impact of culture on beliefs, behaviors, practices, and language related to health." The Commission added that there is a deep and inseparable relationship between cultural competence and the quality of health care.[7] Graduates of Morehouse School of Medicine are in tune with these ideas, because such concepts are taught as part of the institution's curriculum. Louis Sullivan said:

> This school has had an impact in many ways—certainly academically, in terms of the percentage and the number of minority physicians. But in a larger sense, we are helping to change the South in many ways in terms of race relations, the achievements of the Black community, how Whites relate to Blacks, and how Blacks view themselves and their institutions.[8]

Morehouse School of Medicine rode a tide of improving race relations and, through its contributions, pushed this momentum forward.

In addition to its commitment to excellence in patient care, Morehouse also excels in teaching, learning, and research. The school has graduated many PhDs who pursue research and teaching careers at medical schools and universities across the country. The school also offers master's degrees in public health and research technologies. In Sullivan's words, "a faculty that doesn't do research is not a vibrant faculty." With this in mind, those at Morehouse have enthusiastically pursued research and sponsored research opportunities since the institution's creation.[9] The school has several prominent research institutes, including the Neuroscience Institute, directed by Peter MacLeish. This institute was the first of its kind at a Black college, and it was so successful that the National Institutes of Health sponsored similar programs at 18 other Black colleges, based on Morehouse's success. The

Atlanta-based medical school also boasts a Cardiovascular Research Institute, the Satcher Health Leadership Institute, and the Institute on Health Disparities. Although Morehouse is relatively small in comparison with other U.S. medical schools, by the National Institutes of Health's measure of research dollars per faculty member, it is in the top quartile.[10] In addition, four of the current or former administrative leaders of the institution have been elected to the Institute of Medicine: Louis W. Sullivan, David Satcher, Eve J. Higginbotham, and Gary Gibbons (director of the Cardiovascular Research Institute). On a per capita basis, this amounts to more Institute of Medicine members than any other medical school.[11] Despite this attention to research, the medical school has not lost sight of its primary mission of teaching and community outreach, in contrast to what many other medical schools have done in their push to obtain research dollars.[12]

As a leader in both research and clinical practice, Morehouse is significant in the way it connects African Americans to the sciences. A number of factors have alienated Black Americans from the physical sciences, biology, and medicine—fields that are a critical part of our technologically based society. First, a lack of educational opportunity has limited Blacks' access to these fields, which require many years of study to master. Equally important is the lack of trust many African Americans feel toward the systems that promote medical science and technology. Incidents like the notorious Tuskegee experiment have tainted science in the minds of African Americans, giving them the impression that it is another tool for racial exploitation.[13] Morehouse School of Medicine, however, brings Black Americans back to the center of scientific exploration and practice, making them aware of its benefits and their role in moving it forward.

Public health is an area where Morehouse has taken a lead role. According to Louis Sullivan: "We have helped to emphasize the need for public health measures to improve the health of our population. By that I mean bringing the resources to the issue of public health."[14] For example, the institution has helped to raise the level of consciousness concerning the epidemic of HIV/ AIDS in Black communities, decreasing the stigma around the disease and saving lives. As mentioned earlier, the medical school hosted HIV/AIDS clinics in Atlanta and also worked in several African countries to educate people about the problem.

HIV/AIDS education is one of many ways in which Morehouse School of Medicine has stayed close to its mission of serving the public. This mission is perhaps the school's greatest strength and an area where Morehouse sets an example for other institutions of higher learning. The medical school's founders identified a need that was not being met at any other institution. They went about addressing that need in a very single-minded way, explaining it carefully and eloquently to potential supporters, collaborators, and even detractors. Because of their clear-cut approach, the medical school leadership was able to win support in many corners of American society, including the highest echelons of government. Hugh Gloster knew he would have a sympathetic ear in then president Jimmy Carter, who was eager to change the racial climate and give more opportunities to Blacks. Louis Sullivan may not have known what to expect when he approached George and Barbara Bush for support; however, his persuasive and enthusiastic explanation of what Morehouse was about clearly won the day. Moreover, the medical school leadership cast a wide net in its search for support, counting people like Sam Nunn and Herman Talmadge as friends even though their pasts did not recommend them for the role. As noted, the years following the civil rights movement were a time of pragmatism, and those at the top at Morehouse understood that politicians who earlier shunned the Black community now needed their support.

Another area in which the Morehouse leadership excelled was establishing social connections within its most valuable support base: Black physicians in Atlanta and elsewhere, graduates of Morehouse College, and prominent members of the Atlanta community at large. These constituencies were critical, because they provided credibility, financial assistance, and a source of trained professionals to help staff the institution. The Morehouse leadership paid ample attention to this support base, holding gatherings in their own homes and one-on-one meetings, and going out to churches and other community organizations to drum up interest in the medical school. They did not limit themselves to the Black community—locally or nationally—in making use of social connections. White Atlanta medical leaders such as Charles Hatcher, whose sympathies for Black medical education were well known, were also invited to the table. In fundraising for the fledgling school, Gloster, Sullivan, and others were both fearless and strategic. They understood that the climate was right for strong support from the federal government as well as from state sources. However, knowing the history of Black colleges and the stigma that they sometimes carried as "outsider" institutions, Morehouse School of Medicine sought the backing of leaders of local philanthropies, especially the Woodruff Foundation and the Coca-Cola Corporation. Founding a new medical school is a daunting task, but the Morehouse leadership took the right steps. They stood by their mission, garnered cooperation from varied sources, and rooted their institution in its community. The medical school's founding offers a blueprint for the development of educational institutions.

An area of greater difficulty in the school's history was its leadership succession. Here, Morehouse School of Medicine's experience mirrors the missteps of many other institutions as they grow from an idea to a reality. As a new organization, Morehouse needed strong personalities to promote its development—people who held fast even in the face of opposition. One such person was Hugh Gloster, who saw the need for the medical school when others did not and pursued the idea doggedly when others felt the obstacles were too great. Another was Louis Sullivan, who brought strong research credentials and tenacious negotiating skills to bear in building the institution. As often happens with founder-driven institutions, though, the founder held on too long, making it difficult for new leadership to have an impact on the medical school. A series of missteps led to one new president being forced out in a very public confrontation, and another being put in the awkward position of having to remove the founder from the board. The first of these leaders, James Gavin, undermined his own effectiveness by not bringing in his own transition team to Morehouse School of Medicine. In the minds of many, however, the way in which his tenure ended was not entirely fair. The second, David Satcher, guided the institution through treacherous straits, but one wonders why he did not place his name in the hat for the presidency, and, if he had, what would have been the result. Although Morehouse's dedicated faculty and staff were able to carry the institution through tumultuous times, these leadership crises did untold damage, and divisions still exist in the medical school and its surrounding community.

Future Challenges

Morehouse School of Medicine faces several challenges in the coming years. The most pressing is the status of its clinical training site, Grady Memorial Hospital. Since the 1980s, health care costs have more than doubled (rising on average about 4.5% per year since 1993), and reimbursement rates for both governmental medical programs (Medicare and Medicaid) and private insurers have plummeted. Meanwhile, the number of uninsured and underinsured patients has continued to grow rapidly. Nearly 50 percent of the patients at Grady Hospital have no insurance. On top of this, financial support for Grady Hospital from Fulton and DeKalb counties has fallen in recent years. For example, in 1999 the two counties gave the hospital $22 million less than they did in 1993. Despite this huge drop in funding and an erroneous public perception that the hospital is badly managed, Grady has run a highly cost-effective ship relative to its peer institutions. According to a 1993 management review, Grady spent 40 percent less in operating expenses per admission than similar providers, while its public subsidy was 48 percent lower. And most of the uninsured patients at Grady Hospital live in Fulton and DeKalb counties, which have the highest rates in the state for trauma, HIV/AIDS, tuberculosis, and many other high-cost illnesses.[15]

In 2006 Grady Hospital was in financial and leadership turmoil, facing a loss of $21 million, and it was under pressure to make major cuts, including slashing hundreds of jobs and dismantling several programs. After a year of leadership changes, including a new Board of Trustees, and after the hospital hired consultants to give advice on cleaning up the financial problems, the Robert Woodruff Foundation made a $200 million grant to the public hospital to help revive it.[16] On July 21, 2008, the new Grady Hospital board named Michael Young, the former leader of Erie County Medical Center in New York State, as the new CEO. Although Grady is turning its situation around, the atmosphere of instability presents problems for Morehouse. Learning the practice of medicine is challenging for any student, but even more so for Morehouse students learning in Grady's under-resourced environment. The hospital's financial woes have also led to a situation in which both Morehouse and Emory have not been paid for their contributions to the medical care provided at Grady. Despite these challenges, those affiliated with Morehouse School of Medicine and Grady Memorial Hospital hope that a positive relationship will continue and that Morehouse physicians will keep providing much-needed primary care to the low-income and minority populations of Atlanta.[17]

Another challenge for the Atlanta-based medical school is in the area of private fundraising. In spite of its status as a private medical school, Morehouse School of Medicine has relied heavily on both state and federal funding. In the coming years, the institution will need to draw more from private sources, including corporations, foundations, and individuals. As its alumni become more affluent, they must be brought into the medical school's giving process. Alumni sustain institutions, and foundations and corporate donors look to their financial contributions as an indication of the strength and value of an institution's educational program.[18] Morehouse School of Medicine is poised to engage its alumni, who are committed and loyal to their alma mater. With their help and the support of private donors, the medical school will consider an endowment campaign to sustain the institution in the long term.

One could argue that establishing a predominantly Black medical school allows existing White medical schools to shirk their responsibilities in terms of educating African American doctors and reaching out to urban and rural Black communities. However, supporters of Morehouse School of Medicine, as well as African American doctors in the Atlanta community, argue that the magnitude of the need for Black doctors cannot be met by Black medical schools alone. Historically White medical schools still need to provide more access to Black students. For instance, in the first decade of this century, some 1,500 African Americans have entered medical school every year, yet Black medical schools have had enough space for only about 300 of these students. The majority of Black students go to historically White institutions.[19] Morehouse School of Medicine is one choice African Americans have among a larger group of American medical schools. Some students may desire a research-oriented education, whereas others want to pursue a career in primary care. The beauty of medical education in the United States is that schools of medicine are not cookie-cutter images of each other.

Born out of a need for more African American and other minority doctors, begun in a trailer on the Morehouse College campus, and led by a host of ambitious individuals dedicated to primary care, public health, and serving the underserved, Morehouse School of Medicine has flourished and prospered over its first three decades. The institution has overcome skepticism, competition for support, and a turbulent period in its leadership to emerge as a successful and vital contributor to medical education in the United States. Today, the value of the Morehouse School of Medicine cannot be understated. According to a recent report titled *Minorities in Medical Education*, issued by the Council on Graduate Medical Education, "the rapidly changing demographic composition of the U.S. population compels a re-evaluation of who will be the physician of the future, and how that physician's background and sociocultural experiences will prepare him or her for understanding each patient's needs."[20] Moreover, the report argues that "when physicians and patients differ with respect to race, ethnicity, language, religion, and values, ensuring fair, equitable, and culturally sensitive care is more challenging."[21] Morehouse has built a national reputation for itself, instilling cultural sensitivity in all its students, regardless of their racial or ethnic backgrounds. As such, it is vital that the institution continue to grow and to thrive.

Alumni Carrying Out the Mission

Morehouse School of Medicine's unique mission is to provide primary care and serve the underprivileged and underserved. Many of the institution's alumni exemplify this mission. Remarkably, given its size and youth in terms of medical schools, the institution has many notable alumni who have made meaningful contributions across the nation and the world in the areas of primary care for the poor, HIV/AIDS research and programs in Africa, medical education, and government service.

Regina M. Benjamin

Regina M. Benjamin is perhaps the quintessential example of a Morehouse graduate's commitment to medicine for the underserved, having recently both won a MacArthur "Genius" Award and been confirmed as Surgeon General of the U. S. Public Health Service. Benjamin was in the second class of students, attending when the medical school was only a two-year institution. She graduated in 1982. She finished her third and fourth years at the University of Alabama at Birmingham, earning her MD in 1984.[1] Prior to attending the Morehouse medical school, Benjamin attended Xavier University in New Orleans, which has a distinguished record for sending African Americans on to successfully complete medical school.[2] In fact, in the past decade more graduates from this small school have then gone to medical school than those from any other college or university in the country.[3]

Upon completing her medical residency in family practice in Macon at the Medical Center of Central Georgia, she opened an office in Bayou la Batre, Alabama, a small shrimp-fishing village along the Gulf Coast, the region in which she was born and raised.[4] Of note, Bayou la Batre is home to roughly 2,500 residents, mostly working poor. The low-paying jobs available to them typically do not provide health insurance.[5] In an effort to keep her doctor's office open for the surrounding community—an absolute necessity, as she has been the only family doctor in Bayou la Batre since 1990—Benjamin would take on extra work in local emergency rooms and nursing homes.[6] According to Mary Kay Murphy, Morehouse School of Medicine's associate vice president for institutional advancement, when patients could not pay the small fee that she charged, Benjamin accepted barter in the form of seafood, chickens, fruits, and vegetables. This barter

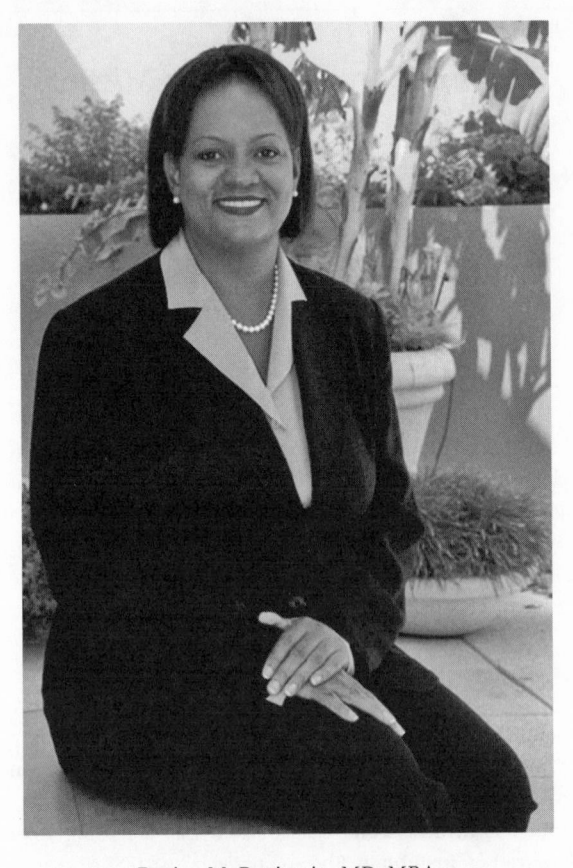

Regina M. Benjamin, MD, MBA.

system maintained the patients' dignity by allowing them to offer something in exchange for Benjamin's services.[7] When Hurricane George struck the Gulf Coast and destroyed her office in 1998, she cared for patients out of the back of her Ford pickup truck.[8] Meanwhile, local volunteers helped to rebuild the office. Sadly, it burned down the day before it was to reopen.[9] Benjamin nonetheless persevered.

She returned to school yet again, earning an MBA from Tulane University in 1991.[10] After obtaining more management training, she converted her private practice into a rural health clinic.[11] Suffering yet another tragedy, this clinic was destroyed by Hurricane Katrina in 2005 and again by another fire later that same year. Benjamin rebuilt the clinic with funds she raised around the nation and was able to continue providing her patients with quality care.[12]

In 1995 Benjamin was elected to the American Medical Association's (AMA) Board of Trustees. When she earned this honor, she was both the first doctor under age 40 and the first African American woman to be elected to the board. She also served as president of the AMA's Education and Research Foundation and on its Council on Ethical and Judicial Affairs.[13] In 1998 Benjamin was awarded the Nelson Mandela Award for Health and Human Rights, and in 2002 she was elected by her peers to the presidency of the State of Alabama's Medical Association, making her the first African American female president of a state medical society in the United States.[14]

For her service and dedication to primary care, Benjamin has received many honors and awards, as well as invitations to serve on national boards pertaining to her areas of expertise and service. She is a Fellow of the American Academy of Family Physicians and served on the boards of the Kaiser Commission on Medicaid and the Uninsured, Catholic Health East, the Federation of State Medical Boards, the Alabama Board of Medical Examiners, the Alabama State Committee of Public Health, the Alabama Rural Health Association, Leadership Alabama, the Mobile Area Red Cross, Mercy Medical, and United Way of Mobile. She was also a trustee of Birmingham Southern University, Morehouse School of Medicine, and Florida A&M University.[15]

In Alabama, Regina Benjamin was a member of the Governor's Health Care Reform Task Force and the Governor's Task Force on Children's Health, and she also served as vice president of the Governor's Commission on Aging. In addition, she is a former board member of Physicians for Human Rights and has spent time doing missionary work in Honduras.[16]

As a result of her development of a rural nonprofit clinic in the low-income community of Bayou la Batre and her constant dedication to patient care without regard to their ability to pay for services, *Time* magazine named Regina Benjamin as one of the "Nation's 50 Future Leaders Age 40 and Under."[17] She was also named "Woman of the Year" by *CBS This Morning*, featured in a *New York Times* article entitled "Angel in a White Coat," and dubbed "Person of the Week" on *ABC World News Tonight*.[18] She was featured on the December 1999 cover of *Clarity* magazine, and she has been the recipient of both the "National Caring Award" (inspired by Mother Teresa) in 2000, and of the papal honor "Pro Ecclesia et Pontifice" from Pope Benedict XVI.[19] In 2008 Dr. Benjamin was given the Award of Honor by the American Hospital Association "in recognition of her outstanding contributions to improving the health status of communities and the nation."[20] That same year Benjamin received a $500,000 MacArthur "Genius" Award, and was named one of "America's Best Leaders" by *US News and World Report*.[21]

Sam Gulube

Native South African Sam Gulube, another prominent alumnus of Morehouse School of Medicine, served as the personal physician to the former president of South Africa, Thabo Mbeki. He is currently the national medical director of the South African National Blood Service. Gulube received his MD from Morehouse School of Medicine in 1991. After completing postgraduate surgical training at the University of South Florida in Tampa, Gulube returned to South Africa in 1997. Interestingly, Sam Gulube used an alias while a student at the medical school—"David Ndaba." According to Louis Sullivan, Gulube was one of the leaders of a student uprising at the University of Natal in Durban,

South Africa, during apartheid in 1976 and had to escape South Africa to avoid arrest. He changed his name to avoid being discovered by South African government hit squads sent abroad by the apartheid government.[22]

From 2003 to 2006, he served as chief executive officer of the Universal Service Agency of South Africa (USASA), which seeks to provide universal access to technology and communication. During his tenure with the USASA, Gulube worked to increase the availability of telecommunications and other technology to people throughout South Africa—particularly in underserved areas—which, in turn, could be used to promote health education and deliver equitable health care.[23] Under his leadership, the USASA established a partnership with Microsoft that provided the company's software for free to 284 community telecenters, changing the lives of myriad individuals in terms of their access to technology.[24]

In 2006 Gulube resigned his position at USASA to join the South African National Blood Service.[25] As the organization's medical director, a high point of his career was announcing in 2008 that there have been no HIV, hepatitis B or hepatitis C transmissions through donated blood since October 2005.[26] Gulube has held various senior positions with the Medical Research Council of South Africa and the National Department of Health.[27] In 2007 Gulube joined the advisory board of Viral Genetics Inc., which is working to develop HIV/AIDS treatment and prevention products in Africa.[28]

Wayne J. Riley

Wayne J. Riley received his MD from Morehouse School of Medicine in 1993. He currently serves as the tenth president of Meharry Medical College in Nashville, Tennessee. Before stepping into a leadership role at Meharry, Riley was the vice president and vice-dean for health affairs and governmental relations and an associate professor of medicine at Baylor College of Medicine in Houston, Texas. He earned an undergraduate degree in anthropology from Yale University and also holds two master's degrees—one from Tulane University in New Orleans in public health, and an MBA from Rice University in Houston.[29]

In May 2004 Riley received the Ben Taub General Hospital "Physician of the Year" Award "in recognition of his outstanding professional achievements and dedication to employee-physician relationships through the delivery of patient-centered care."[30]

Upon assuming the presidency of Meharry Medical College in 2007, Riley accepted a $1 million donation from Wal-Mart to the college's Center for Women's Health Research to support research on diseases that disproportionately affect minority women—particularly African American women.[31] Riley recently secured an $18 million grant from the Robert Wood Johnson Foundation to establish a center for health policy research at Meharry.

Currently Riley is actively involved in several community service organizations. He was appointed for a three-year term as a director on the Nashville Symphony Association Board of Directors and also serves as a board member of Pinnacle Financial Partners LLC, the Cheekwood Botanical Museum Board of Trust, the Executive Board of Directors

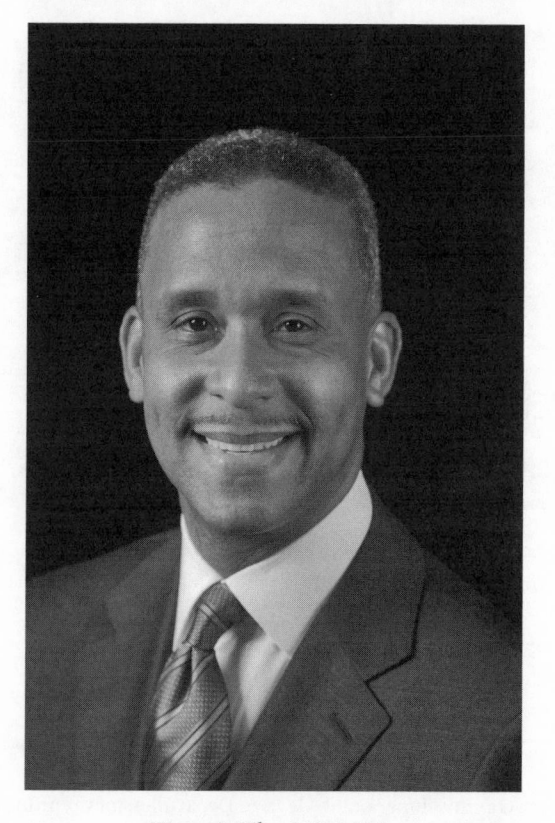

Wayne J. Riley, MD, MBA.

of the Middle Tennessee Council Boy Scouts of America, United Way of Metropolitan Nashville, and the Tennessee Institute of Public Health Board of Directors.[32]

Charlene M. Dewey

Charlene M. Dewey pursued her undergraduate degree at Bradley University, graduating in 1985. She then went on to receive her MD from Morehouse School of Medicine in 1990. While at the Atlanta medical school, Dewey received the Ciba Geigy Award for Academic and Community Leadership and achievement awards from the school's departments of medicine and psychiatry. In 1993 she completed residency training in social internal medicine at the Albert Einstein College of Medicine / Montefiore Medical Center. Dewey then joined the faculty of Baylor College of Medicine in Houston, Texas, as an instructor of medicine. In 2003 the school gave her and her husband, Wayne J. Riley, the Fulbright and Jaworski Faculty Excellence Award for their educational leadership. She also won an award at Baylor in 2006 for her "development of enduring educational materials."[33] Dewey joined the faculty at the Vanderbilt University School of Medicine in

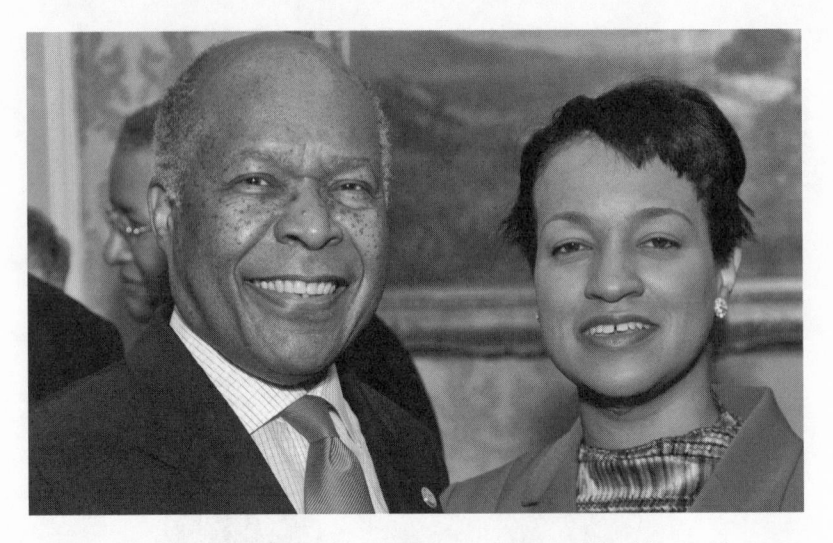

Rhonda Medows (*right*), class of 1986, Georgia Commissioner of Public Health
(2005–2010), with Louis W. Sullivan (*left*). Photograph courtesy of Horace C. Henry.

September 2007. She was recently appointed to the school's Academy of Teaching Excellence and is codirector of the Center for Professional Health.[34]

Rhonda Medows

Rhonda Medows, commissioner of the Georgia Department of Community Health from 2005 to 2010, graduated from Morehouse School of Medicine in 1986. As commissioner, she led a $12.3 billion agency responsible for the purchasing, planning, and regulation of health care for over 2.1 million Georgians. Through her work with the department, she was involved in implementing several major health care initiatives for Georgia's Medicaid, PeachCare Health Insurance Program for Kids, and the State Health Benefit Plan. From 2001 through 2004 she served as Secretary of Florida's Agency for Health Care Administration. She left this position in 2004 to pursue private practice. That same year she joined Specialty Disease Management Services Inc. as a consultant and advisor, later assuming the role of chief medical officer. Medows was also a member of Task Force 6, a task force of the Future of Family Medicine project that created a "financial model that sustains and promotes a thriving New Model of care by focusing on practice reimbursement and health care finances."[35] The Future of Family Medicine aims to "develop a strategy to transform and renew the discipline of family medicine to meet the needs of patients in a changing health care environment."[36]

Medows was a member of the National Governors Association's State Alliance for E-Health, where she served on the Health Information Communication and Data Exchange Taskforce. She was active in efforts to encourage Georgia doctors to employ technology to improve health care, including the use of electronic health records and interactive patient/hospital websites.[37]

In 2008 Medows received an Advocacy Award from the Healthcare Information and Management Systems Society, which honors "leaders who not only believe that health care can be transformed through information technology but also endeavor to make it a reality via national laws, regulations, and public policy."[38] Medows is also active in discussions to improve Medicaid and health care in general for needy patients.[39]

Stephen A. Dawkins

Stephen A. Dawkins graduated from Morehouse School of Medicine in 2000 and currently serves as the medical director at Caduceus Occupational Medicine, having been in this position since 1999. Caduceus is an orthopedic surgery company in Atlanta, Georgia. Before this, Dawkins was the medical director of Sentry Software and of Hospital Occupational Medicine.

Prior to earning his MD, Dawkins received a BS degree in health systems from the Georgia Institute of Technology. He also has an MPH degree from Columbia University. Dawkins is an invited member of the American College of Preventive Medicine, a certified medical review officer, and a member of the American College of Occupational and Environmental Medicine, where he serves on the Committee on Workers' Compensation. According to Mary Kay Murphy, Dawkins has been an active member of the Morehouse School of Medicine alumni for years. He gives motivational speeches and seminars to medical school students, in particular to those at Morehouse.[40]

Jacqueline Holt Grant

Jacqueline Holt Grant graduated with her MD from Morehouse School of Medicine in 1988, and she was one of the first inductees into the school's Alpha Omega Alpha Honor Society.[41] She is now the director of the Southwest Georgia Health District. In this position, she is responsible for 14 counties and serves over 300,000 residents of the state. This impoverished section of Georgia has low median incomes and low high school graduation rates, compared with other districts in the state.[42] To combat the formidable problems of the region, Grant is active in a program called "Hooked on Health," which aims to "lower the burden of chronic disease."[43] The "Hooked on Health" program focuses on smoking cessation, stress reduction, better nutrition, and physical activity, and it offers health information on an interactive website. In 2006 she won an award from Live Healthy Georgia for her efforts in helping to reduce the burden of chronic illness and assisting individuals to lead healthier lives.

Robert S. Kaufmann

Robert S. Kaufmann, a 1986 graduate of Morehouse School of Medicine, is an internal medicine physician at the Kaufmann Clinic in Atlanta, Georgia, which provides primary health care management to adolescent, adult, and geriatric patients. His father, James A. Kaufmann, founded the clinic in 1954. Kaufmann holds an undergraduate degree from the University of Georgia, in addition to his MD.

Along with his role at the clinic, Kaufmann is a clinical assistant professor of medicine at Emory University's School of Medicine, a post he has held since 1993. He is a Fellow of the American College of Physicians. From 1996 to 1997, Kaufmann served as president of Crawford Long Hospital of the Emory University System of Health Care.

In addition to his professional and academic appointments, Kaufmann is a board member of the Alzheimer's Association, a board member of the Atlanta chapter of the National Association for the Advancement of Colored People, and a volunteer with Mercy Mobile Volunteer Physicians. In 1996 he also donated his time to the Volunteer Physicians for Atlanta Paralympic Committee.[44]

Introduction

1. The Commission to End Health Care Disparities, *Unifying Efforts to Achieve Quality Care for All Americans*, Five-Year Summary Report ([Chicago]: AMA [American Medical Association], 2009), 3. See also AMA Council on Science and Public Health, *Ethnic Disparities in Health Care* (Washington, DC: AMA, 2004). The Commission's report quoted it as noting racial and ethnic disparities in "morbidity and mortality from a number of diseases, including heart disease, stroke, cancer, diabetes, asthma and HIV/AIDS" (p. 4).

2. This report is quoted in Commission to End Health Care Disparities, *Unifying Efforts*, 3.

3. Ibid.

4. Fitzhugh Mullan, Candice Chen, Stephen Petterson, Gretchen Kolsky, and Michael Spagnola, "The Social Mission of Medical Education: Ranking the Schools," *Annals of Internal Medicine* 125, no. 12, 804–812.

5. Ibid.

6. This report, "African American Physicians and Organized Medicine, 1846–1968," was also published in the *Journal of the American Medical Association*, vol. 300, no. 3 (2008), 306–313.

7. Ronald M. Davis, speech to the American Medical Association membership, July 30, 2008. See also Ronald M. Davis, "Achieving Racial Harmony for the Benefit of Patients and Communities: Contrition, Reconciliation, and Collaboration," *Journal of the American Medical Association*, vol. 300, no. 3 (2008), 323–325.

8. Davis, speech to the AMA, 2.

9. Ibid.

10. Kevin B. O'Reilly, "AMA Apologizes for Past Inequality against Black Doctors," *American Medical News*, July 28, 2007.

11. Larry Cuban, *How Scholars Trumped Teachers: Change Without Reform in University Curriculum, Teaching, and Research, 1890–1990* (New York: Teachers College Press, 1999), 134.

12. Commission to End Health Care Disparities, *Unifying Efforts*, 3.

13. Ibid.

14. Joseph L. Johnson, "The Supply of Negro Health Personnel-Physicians," *Journal of Negro Education*, vol. 18, no. 3 (Summer 1949), 346–356.

15. Louis W. Sullivan, interview with Marybeth Gasman, Feb. 5, 2008; Louis W. Sullivan, "The School of Medicine at Morehouse College: Status in 1979 and Plans for the Future," *Journal of the Medical Association of Georgia*, vol. 69 (Aug. 1980), 673–674; Abraham Flexner, *Medical Education in the United States and Canada* (New York: Carnegie Foundation, 1910); Darlene Clark Hine, "The Anatomy of Failure: Medical Education Reform and the Leonard Medical School of Shaw University, 1882–1920," *Journal of Negro Education*, vol. 54, no.4 (Autumn 1985), 512–525.

16. Louis W. Sullivan, "The Morehouse School of Medicine: A State of Mind, of Mission, and of Commitment," *Journal of the Medical Association of Georgia*, vol. 72 (July 1983), 490.

17. Ibid.

18. David Satcher, interview with Marybeth Gasman, Apr. 8, 2008; Sullivan, "State of Mind."

19. Cynthia Griggs Fleming, *In the Shadow of Selma: The Continuing Struggle for Civil Rights in the Rural South* (Lanham, MD: Rowman & Littlefield, 2004); J. Mills Thornton, *Dividing Lines: Municipal Politics and the Struggle for Civil Rights in Montgomery, Birmingham, and Selma* (Tuscaloosa: University of Alabama Press, 2002).

20. Fleming, *In the Shadow of Selma*; Thornton, *Dividing Lines*.

21. Alexander Tsesis, *We Shall Overcome: A History of Civil Rights and the Law* (New Haven, CT: Yale University Press, 2008); Robert J. Kaczorowski, *The Politics of Judicial Interpretation: The Federal Courts, Department of Justice, and Civil Rights, 1866–1876* (New York: Fordham University Press, 2005); David J. Garrow, *Protest at Selma: Martin Luther King Jr. and the Voting Rights Act of 1965* (New Haven, CT: Yale University Press, 1980).

22. In 1962, Leroy Johnson was the first African American elected to the Georgia senate since the Reconstruction.

23. Harry G. Lefever, *Undaunted by the Fight: Spelman College and the Civil Rights Museum, 1957–1967* (Macon, GA: Mercer University Press, 2005); David Harmon, *Beneath the Image of the Civil Rights Movement and Race Relations: Atlanta, Georgia, 1946–1981* (New York: Garland, 1996).

24. Bob Short, *Everything Is Pickrick: The Life of Lester Maddox* (Macon, GA: Mercer University Press, 1999); Bruce Galphin, *The Riddle of Lester Maddox* (Atlanta: Camelot, 1968); Lester Maddox, *Speaking Out: The Autobiography of Lester G. Maddox* (Garden City, NJ: Doubleday, 1975); James D. Anderson, *The Education of Blacks in the South, 1865–1930* (Chapel Hill: University of North Carolina Press, 1988); Peter Wallenstein, ed., *Higher Education and the Civil Rights Movement: White Supremacy, Black Southerners, and College Campuses* (Gainesville: University of Florida Press, 2008); Horace T. Ward, *Desegregation of the University of Georgia, Civil Rights Advocacy, and Jurisprudence* (Atlanta: Clark-Atlanta University Press, 2001); Winston A. Grady-Willis, *Challenging U.S. Apartheid: Atlanta and Black Struggles for Human Rights, 1960–1977* (Durham, NC: Duke University Press, 2006); Rhodes Haverty, interview with Marybeth Gasman, Feb. 11, 2009.

25. Janet Abu-Lughod, *Race, Space, and Riots in Chicago, New York, and Los Angeles* (New York: Oxford University Press, 2007); Kevin Mumford, *A History of Race, Rights, and Riots in America* (New York: New York University Press, 2007).

26. Juan Williams, *Thurgood Marshall: American Revolutionary* (New York: Broadway Books, 2000).

27. Michael Eric Dyson, *April 4, 1968: Martin Luther King Jr.'s Death and How It Changed America* (New York: Basic Books, 2008); David J. Garrow, *Bearing the Cross: Martin Luther King Jr. and the Southern Christian Leadership Conference* (New York: W. Morrow, 1986).

28. Short, *Everything Is Pickrick*; Galphin, *Riddle of Lester Maddox*; Maddox, *Speaking Out*.

29. Jimmy Carter, interview with Marybeth Gasman, Sept. 28, 2008.

30. Mullan et al., "Social Mission of Medical Education."

31. Commission to End Health Care Disparities, *Unifying Efforts*.

32. Miriam Komaromy, Kevin Grumbach, Michael Drake, Karen Vranizan, Nicole Lurie, Dennis Keane, and Andrew B. Bindman, "The Role of Black and Hispanic Physicians in Providing Health Care for Underserved Populations," *New England Journal of Medicine*, vol. 334, no. 20 (May 16, 1996), 1305–1310.

Chapter 1 · *African Americans and the Medical Profession*

1. Wilbur H. Watson, *Against the Odds: Blacks in the Profession of Medicine in the United States* (New Brunswick, NJ: Transaction Publishers, 1999).

2. Ibid. See also Werner Sollers, Caldwell Titcomb, and Thomas Underwood, eds., *Blacks at Harvard: A Documentary History of African American Experience at Harvard and Radcliffe* (New York: New York University Press, 2003).

3. Watson, *Against the Odds*. It should be noted that Cleveland is located in the former abolitionist state of Ohio.

4. Ibid.

5. James D. Anderson, *The Education of Blacks in the South, 1865–1930* (Chapel Hill: University of North Carolina Press, 1988); Marybeth Gasman, *Envisioning Black Colleges: A History of the United Negro College Fund* (Baltimore: Johns Hopkins University Press, 2008).

6. Todd L. Savitt, *Race & Medicine in Nineteenth- and Early Twentieth-Century America* (Kent, OH: Kent State University Press, 2007).

7. Christopher Jencks and David Riesman, *The Academic Revolution* (Chicago: University of Chicago Press, 1968), 213.

8. Jencks and Riesman, *Academic Revolution*.

9. Savitt, *Race & Medicine*; Dietrich C. Reitzes and Hekmat Elkhanialy, "Black Physicians and Minority Group Health Care: The Impact of NMF," *Medical Care*, vol. 14, no. 12 (Dec. 1976), 1052–1060.

10. Watson, *Against the Odds*; Rayford Logan, *Howard University: The First Hundred Years, 1867–1967* (New York: New York University Press, 2004).

11. Watson, *Against the Odds*; Clifford L. Muse Jr., "Howard University and the Federal Government During the Presidential Administrations of Herbert Hoover and Franklin D. Roosevelt, 1928–1945," *Journal of Negro History*, vol. 1, no. 4 (1991), 1–20; Logan, *Howard University*.

12. Paul Starr, *The Social Transformation of American Medicine: The Rise of a Sovereign Profession and the Making of a Vast Industry* (New York: Basic Books, 1982).

13. Savitt, *Race & Medicine*, 140.

14. Savitt, *Race & Medicine*; Dietrich C. Reitzes, *Negroes and Medicine* (Cambridge, MA: Harvard University Press, 1958).

15. Watson, *Against the Odds*; Darlene Clark Hine, "The Anatomy of Failure: Medical Education Reform and the Leonard Medical School of Shaw University, 1882–1920," *Journal of Negro Education*, vol. 54, no. 4 (Autumn 1985), 512–525.

16. Savitt, *Race & Medicine*; Clark Hine, "Anatomy of Failure."

17. Savitt, *Race & Medicine*; Anderson, *Education of Blacks*.

18. Savitt, *Race & Medicine*.

19. Ibid. See also Todd L. Savitt, "Lincoln University Medical Department—a Forgotten 19th Century Black Medical School," *Journal of the History of Medicine and Allied Sciences*, vol. 40, no. 1 (1985), 42–65; Horace Mann Bond, *Education for Freedom* (Princeton, NJ: Princeton University Press, 1976).

20. Savitt, *Race & Medicine*; Abraham Flexner, *Medical Education in the United States and Canada* (New York: Arno Press, 1910), 180–181.

21. Savitt, *Race & Medicine*.

22. Ibid. See also Todd L. Savitt, "Four African American Proprietary Medical Schools, 1888–1923," *Journal of the History of Medicine and Allied Sciences*, vol. 55, no. 3 (2000), 203–255.

23. Savitt, *Race & Medicine*, 190.

24. Earl H. Harley, "The Forgotten History of Defunct Black Medical Schools in the 19th and 20th Centuries and the Impact of the Flexner Report," *Journal of the National Medical Association*, vol. 98, no. 9 (2006), 1425–1429; Savitt, *Race & Medicine*.

25. Savitt, *Race & Medicine*; Raymond Fosdick, *Adventures in Giving: The Story of the General Education Board* (New York: Harper & Row, 1962); General Education Board, *The General Education Board: An Account of Its Activities, 1902–1914* (New York: General Education Board, 1915).

26. Starr, *Social Transformation*. For a detailed discussion, see pp. 124–135 of Starr's book.

27. Harley, "Forgotten History."

28. Starr, *Social Transformation*. For a detailed discussion, see pp. 124–135 of Starr's book.

29. Ibid., 117.

30. Ibid.

31. Savitt, *Race & Medicine*, 254.

32. Ibid.

33. James G. Burrow, *American Medical Association: Voice of American Medicine* (Baltimore: Johns Hopkins Press, 1963); Morris Fishbein, *History of the American Medical Association, 1847–1947* (Philadelphia: W. B. Saunders, 1947).

34. Flexner, *Medical Education*, 180–181; Thomas Neville Bonner, *Iconoclast: Abraham Flexner and a Life in Learning* (Baltimore: Johns Hopkins University Press, 2002).

35. Bonner, *Iconoclast*; Flexner, *Medical Education*, 180–181.

36. Larry Cuban, *How Scholars Trumped Teachers: Change without Reform in University Curriculum, Teaching, and Research, 1890–1990* (New York: Teachers College Press, 1999).

37. Jencks and Riesman, *Academic Revolution*.

38. Starr, *Social Transformation*. Starr makes a convincing argument that medical schools faced increased expenses as medicine became more complex, including the need for modern laboratories, libraries, and clinical facilities.

39. Campbell Gibson and Kay Jung, "Historical Census Statistics on Population Totals

by Race, 1790 to 1990," available at www.census.gov. See also Louis W. Sullivan and Ilana Suez Mittman, "The State of Diversity in the Health Professions a Century after Flexner," *Academic Medicine*, vol. 85, no. 2 (Feb. 2010), 246–253.

40. Gibson and Jung, "Historical Census Statistics." See also Sullivan and Mittman, "State of Diversity."

41. Flexner, *Medical Education*, 180–181.

42. Savitt, *Race & Medicine*, 180–181.

43. Ibid., 252.

44. Starr, *Social Transformation*.

45. Savitt, *Race & Medicine*; H. A. Callis, "The Need and Training of Negro Physicians," *Journal of Negro Education*, vol. 4, no. 1 (Jan. 1935), 32–41; Numa P. G. Adams, "Sources of Supply of Negro Health Personnel, Section A: Physicians," *Journal of Negro Education*, vol. 6, no. 3 (July 1937), 468–467; Elijah H. Allen Jr., "A Selected Annotated Bibliography on the Health Education of the Negro," *Journal of Negro Education*, vol. 6, no. 3 (July 1937): 578–581.

46. Savitt, *Race & Medicine*; Logan, *Howard University*; Callis, "Need and Training"; Adams, "Sources of Supply"; Allen, "Selected Annotated Bibliography"; Karen Kruse Thomas, "Dr. Jim Crow: The University of North Carolina, the Regional Medical School for Negroes, and the Desegregation of Southern Medical Education, 1945–1960," *Journal of African American History*, vol. 88, no. 3 (Summer 2003), 223–244.

47. Savitt, *Race & Medicine*.

48. See materials at the Rockefeller Archive Center in Sleepy Hollow, New York; Anderson, *Education of Blacks*; William H. Watkins, *The White Architects of Black Education: Ideology and Power in America, 1865–1954* (New York: Teachers College Press, 2001).

49. Fosdick, *Adventures in Giving*; General Education Board, *General Education Board*.

50. Savitt, *Race & Medicine*, 263.

51. Robert B. Baker, Harriet A. Washington, Ololade Olakanmi, Todd L. Savitt, Elizabeth A. Jacobs, Eddie Hoover, and Matthew K. Wynia, "African American Physicians and Organized Medicine, 1846–1968," *Journal of the American Medical Association*, vol. 300, no. 3 (2008), 306–313; Callis, "Need and Training."

52. John A. Kennedy, "Some Notes on the History of the National Medical Association," *Journal of the National Medical Association*, vol. 25, no. 3 (Aug. 25, 1933), 97–105.

53. Thomas J. Ward, *Black Physicians in the Jim Crow South* (Fayetteville: University of Arkansas Press, 2003).

54. Baker et al., "African American Physicians." See also Kennedy, "Some Notes."

55. Savitt, *Race & Medicine*, 258. See also Flexner, *Medical Education*, 180–181.

56. Flexner, *Medical Education*, 180–181. See also Savitt, *Race & Medicine*.

57. Ibid.

58. Flexner, quoted in Baker et al., "African American Physicians," 304.

59. Baker et al., "African American Physicians" ; Henry H. Hazen, "Twenty-Three Years of Teaching in a Negro Medical School," *Social Forces*, vol. 12, no. 4 (May 1934), 570–575.

60. Joseph L. Johnson, "The Supply of Negro Health Personnel—Physicians," *Journal of Negro Education*, vol. 18, no. 3 (Summer 1949), 346–356.

61. Ward, *Black Physicians*; Bonner, *Iconoclast*.

62. Ward, *Black Physicians.*

63. Johnson, "Supply."

64. Ibid.

65. Andrew A. Sorensen, "Black Americans and the Medical Profession, 1930–1970," *Journal of Negro Education,* vol. 41, no. 4 (Autumn 1972), 337–342; Ward, *Black Physicians.*

66. Sorensen, "Black Americans."

67. Ruth M. Raup and Elizabeth A. Williams, "Negro Students in Medical Education in the United States," *Journal of Medical Education,* vol. 39 (May 1964), 444–450.

68. Ward, *Black Physicians.*

69. Watson, *Against the Odds.*

70. Ibid.

71. Michel P. Richard, "The Negro Physician: Babbitt or Revolutionary?" *Journal of Health and Social Behavior,* vol. 10, no. 4 (Dec. 1969), 265–274.

72. Watson, *Against the Odds.*

73. Ibid., 37. See also Starr, *Social Transformation.*

74. Watson, *Against the Odds*; Baker et al., "African American Physicians."

75. Baker et al., "African American Physicians"; "Naming Selective Colleges That Are Most Preferred by Black Students," *Journal of Blacks in Higher Education,* vol. 30 (Winter 2000/2001), 28.

76. "A Chronology of Significant Events in Duke University's History," Duke University Archives website, http://library.duke.edu/uarchives/history/chronology.html, accessed Oct. 26, 2009; "Legacy of Learning: History," Emory University School of Medicine website, http://www.med.emory.edu/admissions/aboutsomhistory.cfm, accessed Oct. 26, 2009; "History of Vanderbilt University," Vanderbilt University website, www.vanderbilt.edu/about/history/, accessed Oct. 26, 2009.

77. Sorensen, "Black Americans"; Jordan J. Cohen, "The Consequences of Premature Abandonment of Affirmative Action in Medical School Admissions," *Journal of the American Medical Association,* vol. 289, no. 9 (Mar. 5, 2003), 1145; Gail E. Thomas, *The Access and Success of Blacks and Hispanics in U.S. Graduate and Professional Education* (Washington, DC: National Academy Press, 1986), vii, 29.

78. "Naming Selective Colleges."

79. Ibid.

80. Ibid. See also Cohen, "Consequences of Premature Abandonment."

81. "Naming Selective Colleges"; Cohen, "Consequences of Premature Abandonment." Of note, there has also been a decline in the number of White male medical students. Currently, roughly 50 percent of White medical students are women. See also Association of American Medical Schools, Annual Status of Medical Education, report, 2000, Morehouse School of Medicine Archives, Atlanta, Georgia; Laura Perna, Valerie Lundy Wagner, Noah D. Drezner, Marybeth Gasman, Susan Yoon, Enakshi Bose, and Shannon Gary, "The Contributions of Historically Black Colleges and Universities to the Preparation of African American Women for STEM Careers: A Case Study," *Research in Higher Education,* vol. 50, no. 1 (2009), 1–23.

82. Leroy Davis, *A Clashing of the Soul: John Hope and the Dilemma of African American Leadership and Black Higher Education in the Early Twentieth Century* (Athens: University of

Georgia Press, 1998); Vida L. Avery, "A Fateful Hour in Black Higher Education: The Creation of the Atlanta University System," PhD diss., Georgia State University, 2003.

83. Louis W. Sullivan, interview with Marybeth Gasman, Jan. 10, 2008; Davis, *Clashing of the Soul*; Avery, "A Fateful Hour."

84. Asa G. Yancey Sr., interview with Marybeth Gasman, May 13, 2008; Davis, *Clashing of the Soul*; Avery, "A Fateful Hour."

85. Sullivan, interview with Marybeth Gasman, Jan. 10, 2008; Davis, *Clashing of the Soul*; Avery, "A Fateful Hour."

Chapter 2 · Birth of a Medical School

1. Thomas Jarrett to John Z. Bowers, President, Josiah W. Macy Jr. Foundation, Feb. 10, 1970, Morehouse School of Medicine Archives, Atlanta, Georgia. See also Task Force for Physician Manpower, *Physician Manpower in Georgia: Report of the Task Force for Physician Manpower to the Georgia Comprehensive Health Planning Council* (Atlanta: Office of Comprehensive Health Planning, Georgia Department of Public Health, 1967).

2. Coordinating Council on Medical Education, "Physician Manpower and Distribution: The Primary Care Physician," *Journal of the American Medical Association*, vol. 233, no. 8 (Aug. 25, 1975), 880–881. Federal manpower reports were also released in 1957 and 1966. In addition, see Departmental Committee on Higher Education, U.S. Office of Education, "Manpower Needs and Supply," Staff Paper No. 3, 1957; Daniel Patrick Moynihan, "The Impact on Manpower Development and Employment of Youth," in *Universal Higher Education*, ed. Earl James McGrath (New York: McGraw-Hill, 1966), 65–78. For a recent discussion of education in the professions and the impact of the manpower reports, see Lara K. Couturier, "Debating Access to the Professions, 1940–1980," paper presented at the History of Education Society's annual meeting, Philadelphia, Pennsylvania, October 22–25, 2009.

3. Robert B. Baker, Harriet A. Washington, Ololade Olakanmi, Todd L. Savitt, Elizabeth A. Jacobs, Eddie Hoover, and Matthew K. Wynia, "African American Physicians and Organized Medicine, 1846–1968," *Journal of the American Medical Association*, vol. 300, no. 3 (2008), 306–313; Frank Bane, *Physicians for a Growing America: Report of the Surgeon General's Consultant Group on Medical Education*, Publication No. R709 (Washington, DC: U.S. Public Health Service, Department of Health, Education, and Welfare, 1959).

4. Bane, *Physicians*.

5. Ibid. For a general overview of the status of the professions, see also Nathan O. Hatch, ed., *The Professions in American History* (Notre Dame, IN: University of Notre Dame Press, 1988); Bruce A. Kimball, *The "True Professional Ideal" in America: A History* (Cambridge, MA: Blackwell, 1992).

6. Paul Starr, *The Social Transformation of American Medicine: The Rise of a Sovereign Profession and the Making of a Vast Industry* (New York: Basic Books, 1982). See especially 364–365 for a detailed discussion of the "doctor shortage" projected for the 1960s and 1970s.

7. Bane, *Physicians*.

8. Fry Consultants, "A Study of the Feasibility of a Two-Year Medical School at Atlanta University," Jan. 8, 1971.

9. Ibid., 4.

10. Ibid.; Task Force for Physician Manpower, *Physician Manpower in Georgia*; Karen Kruse Thomas, "Dr. Jim Crow: The University of North Carolina, the Regional Medical School for Negroes, and the Desegregation of Southern Medical Education, 1945–1960," *Journal of African American History*, vol. 88, no. 3 (Summer 2003), 223–244.

11. Bureau of the Census, U.S. Department of Commerce, "Intercensal Estimates of the Total Resident Population of States: 1960 to 1970," www.census.gov/popest/archives/1980s/st6070ts.txt.; Asa G. Yancey Sr., "Negroes in Medicine: A Surgeon Looks at Leaders in the Years of Black Emergence in American Medicine," *Medicine at Emory*, vol. 8 (1970), 12–18; Georgia Department of Public Health, "1969 Statistical Abstract of the United States," Morehouse School of Medicine Archives.

12. Fry Consultants, "Study of the Feasibility."

13. Thomas J. Ward, *Black Physicians in the Jim Crow South* (Fayetteville: University of Arkansas Press, 2003).

14. Fry Consultants, "Study of the Feasibility."

15. Ibid. Of note, the first Black medical student at Emory was Hamilton Holmes. He was well known, along with Charlayne Hunter, for having desegregated the University of Georgia in 1961. The hostile atmosphere that these young people experienced in the early 1960s was indicative of the overall racial climate in Georgia. Mobs, including Ku Klux Klan members, appeared on campus to protest the enrollment of both Holmes and Hunter. Much work needed to be done to ensure that Blacks would be welcomed into Georgia higher education overall, including medical education. See also Melissa Kean, *Desegregating Private Higher Education in the South* (Albany: State University of New York Press, 2008).

16. Fry Consultants, "Study of the Feasibility."

17. Christopher Jencks and David Riesman, *The Academic Revolution* (Chicago: University of Chicago Press, 1968), 437. It making the statement regarding Black medical schools, Jencks and Riesman provided a defense of their seemingly racist comment: "The Negro schools were evidently admitting students with lower scores than any but a handful of white schools. . . . The Council on Medical Education of the American Medical Association also reports the percentage of students from each medical school failing state medical board exams each year. In 1965 [there were only two medical schools] with higher failure rates than Meharry and Howard." Jencks and Riesman concluded that the high failure rates reflected the limited ability of the students the medical schools admitted (see p. 437).

18. Task Force for Physician Manpower, *Physician Manpower in Georgia*. See also Fry Consultants, "Study of the Feasibility."

19. Starr, *Social Transformation*.

20. U.S. Bureau of Health Manpower, *Bureau of Health Manpower Report* (Washington, DC: National Institutes of Health, 1970).

21. Yancey, "Negroes in American Medicine."

22. Ibid.; Wayne J. Riley, "Diversity in the Health Professions Matters: The Untold Story of Meharry Medical College," *Journal of Health Care for the Poor and Underserved*, vol. 19 (2008), 331–342.

23. Yancey, "Negroes in American Medicine."

24. Louis W. Sullivan, interview for Morehouse School of Medicine Public Relations

Department, 2007, in the possession of the Public Relations Department, Morehouse School of Medicine, Atlanta, Georgia.

25. Louis W. Sullivan, interview with Marybeth Gasman, Jan. 10, 2008; Yvonne Gloster, interview with Marybeth Gasman, Feb. 10, 2008.

26. Louis W. Sullivan, interview with Marybeth Gasman, Jan. 10, 2008; Clinton Warner, interview with Marybeth Gasman, Feb. 10, 2008; Yvonne Gloster, interview with Marybeth Gasman, Feb. 10, 2008.

27. Louis W. Sullivan, interview with Marybeth Gasman, Jan. 10, 2008; Yvonne Gloster, interview with Marybeth Gasman, Feb. 10, 2008.

28. Clinton Warner, interview with Marybeth Gasman, Feb. 10, 2008; Yvonne Gloster, interview with Marybeth Gasman, Feb. 10, 2008.

29. Louis W. Sullivan, interview for Morehouse School of Medicine Public Relations Department, 2007, Public Relations Department, Morehouse School of Medicine; Rhodes Haverty, interview with Marybeth Gasman, Feb. 11, 2009.

30. Louis W. Sullivan, interview for Morehouse School of Medicine Public Relations Department, 2007, Public Relations Department, Morehouse School of Medicine; Rhodes Haverty, interview with Marybeth Gasman, Feb. 11, 2009.

31. Thomas Jarrett to John Z. Bowers, Feb. 10, 1970, Morehouse School of Medicine Archives.

32. Minutes of the meeting of the Board of Directors, Josiah Macy Jr. Foundation, 1970; as well as minutes of the meeting of the Board of Directors, 1974; minutes of the meeting of the Board of Directors, 1975; minutes of the meeting of the Board of Directors, 1976; all in box 1373, Josiah Macy Jr. Foundation Archives, New York, New York.

33. Thomas Jarrett to John Z. Bowers, Feb. 10, 1970, Morehouse School of Medicine Archives; minutes from the Mar. 7, 1969, board meeting of Atlanta University Center, Morehouse School of Medicine Archives; minutes of the meeting of the Board of Directors, Josiah Macy Jr. Foundation, 1970, box 1373, Josiah Macy Jr. Foundation Archives.

34. Bernard Hallman to President Thomas D. Jarrett, Dec. 14, 1970, Morehouse School of Medicine Archives.

35. Bernard Hallman to Howard Kenney, Jan. 19, 1971, Morehouse School of Medicine Archives.

36. Starr, *Social Transformation*; Larry Cuban, *How Scholars Trumped Teachers: Change without Reform in University Curriculum, Teaching, and Research, 1890–1990* (New York: Teachers College Press, 1999).

37. Fry Consultants, "Proposal for Atlanta University," Dec. 12, 1969.

38. Ibid.

39. Fry Consultants, "Study of the Feasibility."

40. Ibid. For a discussion of medical school curriculum, see Starr, *Social Transformation*; Cuban, *How Scholars Trumped Teachers*.

41. Fry Consultants, "Study of the Feasibility."

42. Ibid.

43. Summary of a conference between Bernard Hallman and Thomas D. Jarrett, July 11, 1968, Morehouse School of Medicine Archives.

44. Cuban, *How Scholars Trumped Teachers.* See especially chapter 5, "How Research Trumped Teaching in History and Medicine."

45. Fry Consultants, "Study of the Feasibility." See also Michael J. Kapsa, *Labor Strife and the Economy in the 1970s: A Decade of Discord* (New York: Garland, 1998).

46. Starr, *Social Transformation,* 384. See also Richard Nixon, "Special Message to the Congress on Health Care," Mar. 2, 1972, American Presidency Project website, www.pres idency.ucsb.edu.

47. Starr, *Social Transformation.*

48. Ibid. See also Richard Nixon, "Statement on Signing the National Sickle Cell Anemia Control Act," May 16, 1972, American Presidency Project website. Nixon's efforts in this area began in 1970.

49. Fry Consultants, "Study of the Feasibility."

50. Ibid., 58.

51. James D. Anderson, *The Education of Blacks in the South, 1865–1930* (Chapel Hill: University of North Carolina Press, 1988); Patrick J. Gilpin and Marybeth Gasman, *Charles Spurgeon Johnson: Leadership Beyond the Veil in the Age of Jim Crow* (Albany: State University of New York Press, 2003).

52. Anderson, *Education of Blacks;* Gilpin and Gasman, *Charles Spurgeon Johnson.*

53. Fry Consultants, "Study of the Feasibility," 62.

54. Ibid, 66.

55. Bernard Nelson to Thomas Jarrett and Arthur Richardson, Mar. 16, 1971, Morehouse School of Medicine Archives. The consultants included Robert S. Anderson, Meharry Medical College; Clifford Barger, the American Physiological Society; John Cooper, Association of American Medical Colleges; Howard Kenny, Veterans Administration; and Bernard Nelson, Stanford Medical School.

56. Louis W. Sullivan, interview for Morehouse School of Medicine Public Relations Department, 2007, Public Relations Department, Morehouse School of Medicine; Yvonne Gloster, interview with Marybeth Gasman, Feb. 10, 2008.

57. This sentiment was prevalent among those interviewed for the book.

58. Louis W. Sullivan, interview with Marybeth Gasman, Jan. 10, 2008; Yvonne Gloster, interview with Marybeth Gasman, Feb. 10, 2008.

59. Louis W. Sullivan, interview with Marybeth Gasman, Jan. 10, 2008; Yancey, "Negroes in American Medicine."

60. Louis W. Sullivan, interview with Marybeth Gasman, Jan. 10, 2008. See also institutional data in the Morehouse College Archives, Atlanta, Georgia; Edward Allen Jones, *A Candle in the Dark: A History of Morehouse College* (Atlanta: Judson Press, 1967); Benjamin Brawley, *History of Morehouse College* (New York: Cosimo Classics, 2009).

61. "Naming Selective Colleges That Are Most Preferred by Black Students," *Journal of Blacks in Higher Education,* vol. 30 (Winter 2000/2001), 28; "U.S. Medical Schools and Applicants" data for 1969 [no longer available], Association of American Medical Colleges website, www.aamc.org.

62. William A. Bennett, interview with Marybeth Gasman, May 19, 2009. See the Morehouse College collection, Library of Congress, Washington, D.C., for information on the federal government's role in establishing the medical school.

63. William A. Bennett, interview with Marybeth Gasman, May 19, 2009.

64. William A. Bennett, interview with Marybeth Gasman, May 19, 2009. This story was also retold by Yvonne Gloster, interview with Marybeth Gasman, Feb. 10, 2008.

65. Louis W. Sullivan, interview with Marybeth Gasman, Jan. 10, 2008; Yvonne Gloster, interview with Marybeth Gasman, Feb. 10, 2008; William A. Bennett, interview with Marybeth Gasman, May 19, 2009.

66. Yvonne Gloster, interview with Marybeth Gasman, Feb. 10, 2008; Jones, *Candle in the Dark.* For a detailed discuss of the Black college presidents' response to the *Brown v. Board of Education* decision, see Marybeth Gasman, *Envisioning Black Colleges: A History of the United Negro College Fund* (Baltimore: Johns Hopkins University Press, 2008).

67. Louis W. Sullivan, interview with Marybeth Gasman, Jan. 7, 2008; Vida L. Avery, "A Fateful Hour in Black Higher Education: The Creation of the Atlanta University System," PhD diss., Georgia State University, 2003.

68. Resolution made at a special meeting of the Atlanta University Board of Trustees, Aug. 12, 1977, 1, Morehouse School of Medicine Archives.

69. Starr, *Social Transformation.*

70. William A. Bennett, interview with Marybeth Gasman, May 19, 2009.

71. William A. Bennett, interview with Marybeth Gasman, May 19, 2009; Yvonne Gloster, interview with Marybeth Gasman, Feb. 10, 2008.

72. William A. Bennett, interview with Marybeth Gasman, May 19, 2009.

73. Laura Perna, Valerie Lundy Wagner, Noah D. Drezner, Marybeth Gasman, Susan Yoon, Enakshi Bose, and Shannon Gary, "The Contributions of Historically Black Colleges and Universities to the Preparation of African American Women for STEM Careers: A Case Study," *Research in Higher Education,* vol. 50, no. 1 (2009), 1–23.

74. Florence M. Read, *The Story of Spelman College* (Princeton, NJ: Princeton University Press, 1961); Beverly Guy-Sheftall, "Black Women and Higher Education: Spelman and Bennett Colleges Revisited," in "The Impact of Black Women in Education: An Historical Overview," special issue, *Journal of Negro Education,* vol. 51, no. 3 (Summer 1982), 278–287.

75. Marybeth Gasman, "Perceptions of Black College Presidents: Sorting Through Stereotypes and Reality to Gain a Complex Picture," *American Education Research Journal* (forthcoming, 2011).

76. Atlanta University Board of Trustee minutes, Nov. 1975, Robert W. Woodruff Library, Atlanta University Center, Atlanta, Georgia; Louis W. Sullivan, interview with Marybeth Gasman, Jan. 11, 2008. This story was also recalled by Yvonne Gloster, interview with Marybeth Gasman, Feb. 10, 2008.

77. Atlanta University Board of Trustee minutes, Nov. 1975, Woodruff Library, Atlanta University Center; Louis W. Sullivan, interview with Marybeth Gasman, Jan. 11, 2008. See also Yvonne Gloster, interview with Marybeth Gasman, Feb. 10, 2008.

78. Resolution made at a special meeting of the Atlanta University Board of Trustees, Aug. 12, 1977, 4, Morehouse School of Medicine Archives.

79. Louis W. Sullivan, interview with Marybeth Gasman, Mar. 12, 2009; Yvonne Gloster, interview with Marybeth Gasman, Feb. 10, 2008; Jones, *Candle in the Dark;* Brawley, *History of Morehouse College.*

80. Fry Consultants, "Study of the Feasibility," annotated copy in the Woodruff Library, Atlanta University Center.

81. Marybeth Gasman, "Truth, Generalizations, and Stigmas: An Analysis of the Media's Coverage of Morris Brown College and Black Colleges Overall," *Review of Black Political Economy*, vol. 34, no.2 (2007), 111–135.

82. The Morehouse College campaign is discussed in detail in Marybeth Gasman and Noah Drezner, "A Maverick in the Field: The Oram Group and Fundraising in the Black College Community During the 1970s," *History of Education Quarterly*, vol. 49, no. 4 (2009), 465–500. For a discussion of the difficulties for Black colleges in the 1970s, see Gasman, *Envisioning Black Colleges*. See also Yvonne Gloster, interview with Marybeth Gasman, Feb. 10, 2008.

83. Yvonne Gloster, interview with Marybeth Gasman, Feb. 10, 2008.

84. Louis W. Sullivan, interview for Morehouse School of Medicine Public Relations Department, 2007, Public Relations Department, Morehouse School of Medicine; Yvonne Gloster, interview with Marybeth Gasman, Feb. 10, 2008.

85. Yvonne Gloster, interview with Marybeth Gasman, Feb. 10, 2008. See also Jones, *Candle in the Dark*.

86. James Story, interview with Marybeth Gasman, Mar. 24, 2008.

87. Yvonne Gloster, interview with Marybeth Gasman, Feb. 10, 2008.

88. Asa G. Yancey Sr., interview with Marybeth Gasman, May 13, 2008.

89. Rhodes Haverty, interview with Marybeth Gasman, Feb. 11, 2009. Several national reports, to be discussed later in this chapter, confirm Haverty's assertions.

90. Rhodes Haverty, interview with Marybeth Gasman, Feb. 11, 2009. See also Clarence Stone, *Regime Politics: Governing Atlanta, 1946–1988* (Lawrence: University Press of Kansas, 1989).

91. Louis W. Sullivan, interview with Marybeth Gasman, Mar. 10, 2008; Rhodes Haverty, interview with Marybeth Gasman, Feb. 11, 2009.

92. Louis W. Sullivan, interview with Marybeth Gasman, Mar. 10, 2008.

93. Rhodes Haverty, interview with Marybeth Gasman, Feb. 11, 2009.

94. Joe Frank Harris, interview with Marybeth Gasman, July 17, 2008. A review of newspaper articles written about Black colleges and Morehouse during the years of the "medical idea" resulted in very few negative stories.

95. Gasman, *Envisioning Black Colleges*.

96. Peter Wallenstein, ed., *Higher Education and the Civil Rights Movement: White Supremacy, Black Southerners, and College Campuses* (Gainesville: University Press of Florida, 2008).

97. Gasman, *Envisioning Black Colleges*; Wallenstein, *Higher Education*.

98. Prior to the *Brown v. Board of Education* decision, the NAACP had staged a carefully planned series of legal battles against Jim Crow education at the graduate school level. In each of these cases, a Black graduate applicant challenged the notion of "separate but equal education." Although Southern states claimed that a Black student could receive an equal education in any field in a separate institution, this was clearly not the case. A Black student wanting to be educated in law, for example, might be sent to another state or made to attend a makeshift "law school" that was created solely for the purpose of compliance and

without any real intent to provide equal education. The first case, in 1938, involved Lloyd Gaines, a Black high school valedictorian who wanted to attend the University of Missouri Law School. When the law school discovered that Gaines was Black, they denied him admission but offered to pay his tuition in another state. In this instance the Court declared that states must either furnish separate and equal educational institutions within the respective state or admit Blacks to the all-White institutions. In effect, *Gaines* called for the provision of an equal education for all of a state's residents. Two additional, yet equally important cases were *Sipuel v. Board of Regents* (1948) and *Sweatt v. Painter* (1950). In the first of these legal challenges, Ada Sipuel had applied to the University of Oklahoma law school and was denied admission based on her race. With the help of the NAACP, Sipuel sued the state and the case eventually reached the U.S. Supreme Court. Based on the Fourteenth Amendment, the Court held that states must provide equal graduate education for Blacks. At first, however, the ruling did not specify how that education was to be provided. Thus, rather than admitting Ada Sipuel to the University of Oklahoma, the state's Board of Regents roped off an area in the state capitol building, designated the area as the "Negro law school," and hired three Black lawyers to serve as the faculty. Eventually, the U.S. Supreme Court decided that this practice was unconstitutional, and Ada Sipuel was allowed to enroll at the University of Oklahoma. The *Sweatt v. Painter* case involved Heman Sweatt, a Black man who applied for admission to the law school at the University of Texas in 1946. Citing the fact that it was a segregated institution, the school rejected Sweat's application. With the assistance of NAACP attorneys, Sweatt sued the university. Although he lost his legal suit at the state level, the U.S. Supreme Court, finding that equal education had been denied, forced the University of Texas law school and the institution's graduate school to open its doors to all students, regardless of race, in 1950. This case, in particular, was a vital predecessor to *Brown v. Board*, because in it the Court unanimously decided that "separate but equal" was not equal. Notably, the Court declared in these decisions that the states not only had an obligation to provide graduate education for Blacks, but that this education must replicate the intellectual level experienced by Whites. These legal challenges established the role of the environment (e.g. the facilities, traditions, and faculty) in the student's experience at a college or university. In order to receive an equal education, a student not only needed to learn the same material, but also be supported in the same way by the institution doing the teaching. Since, in most instances, this could only be achieved by sending Blacks to the same schools as Whites, these decisions made it almost inevitable that segregation would be overturned. See Missouri ex rel. Gaines v. Canada, Registrar of the University of Missouri, et al., 305 U.S. 337 (1938); Sipuel v. Board of Regents, 332 U.S. 631 (1948); Sweatt v. Painter, 339 U.S. 629 (1950); McLaurin v. Oklahoma State Regents, 339 U.S. 637 (1950). For a deeper understanding of these cases, see Michael Klarman, *From Jim Crow to Civil Rights: The Supreme Court and the Struggle for Racial Equality* (New York: Oxford University Press, 2003); Mark Tushet, *NAACP's Legal Strategy against Segregated Education, 1925–1950* (Chapel Hill: University of North Carolina Press, 1987).

99. Marybeth Gasman, Benjamin Baez, and Caroline Sotello Turner, eds., *Understanding Minority-Serving Institutions* (Albany: State University of New York, 2008).

100. "North Carolina Central University School of Law Profile [2009–2010 class profile]," North Carolina Central University School of Law website, www.nccu.edu/law/.

101. James Story, interview with Marybeth Gasman, Mar. 24, 2008.

102. Fry Consultants, "Study of the Feasibility," 61.

103. Ibid., 62.

104. James Story, interview with Marybeth Gasman, Mar. 24, 2008. This sentiment was confirmed by the majority of those interviewed for this book, including Andrew Young.

105. James Story, interview with Marybeth Gasman, Mar. 24, 2008; Rhodes Haverty, interview with Marybeth Gasman, Feb. 11, 2009; Asa G. Yancey Sr., interview with Marybeth Gasman, May 13, 2009; Louis W. Sullivan, interview with Marybeth Gasman, Mar. 10, 2008; Joe Frank Harris, interview with Marybeth Gasman, July 17, 2008.

106. Charles Hatcher, interview with Marybeth Gasman, July 23, 2009.

107. Louis W. Sullivan, interview with Marybeth Gasman, Mar. 12, 2009; Charles Hatcher, interview with Marybeth Gasman, July 23, 2009. Others who were interviewed for this book also alluded to this notion, but declined to have the comments attributed to them.

108. Charles Hatcher, interview with Marybeth Gasman, July 23, 2009.

109. Charles Hatcher, interview with Marybeth Gasman, July 23, 2009.

110. Louis W. Sullivan, interview with Marybeth Gasman, Jan. 11, 2008; Charles Hatcher, interview with Marybeth Gasman, July 23, 2009.

111. Yancey, "Negroes in American Medicine."

112. William G. Bowen and Derek Bok, *The Shape of the River: The Long-Term Consequences of Considering Race in College and University Admissions* (Princeton, NJ: Princeton University Press, 1998).

113. "Morehouse Begins New Era," *Atlanta Constitution*, Sept. 11, 1978, 1A; William A. Bennett, interview with Marybeth Gasman, May 19, 2009. The Bureau of Health Manpower was a part of the National Institutes of Health at the time.

114. Morehouse School of Medicine, "A Short History," unpublished manuscript, May 4, 1988; William A. Bennett, interview with Marybeth Gasman, May 19, 2009.

115. William A. Bennett, interview with Marybeth Gasman, May 19, 2009; Morehouse College statistical files, Morehouse College Archives.

116. Morehouse School of Medicine, "A Short History"; William A. Bennett, interview with Marybeth Gasman, May 19, 2009; James Story, interview with Marybeth Gasman, Mar. 24, 2008.

117. Louis W. Sullivan, interview with Marybeth Gasman, Jan. 11, 2008; James Story, interview with Marybeth Gasman, Mar. 24, 2008; William A. Bennett, interview with Marybeth Gasman, May 19, 2009.

118. James Story, interview with Marybeth Gasman, Mar. 24, 2008; William A. Bennett, interview with Marybeth Gasman, May 19, 2009; Nerimiah Emmett, interview with Marybeth Gasman, Mar. 24, 2008.

119. William A. Bennett, interview, May 19, 2009. Bennett's role is supported by myriad documents in the Morehouse College of Medicine Archives and the Morehouse College Archives. He played an integral part in the early years of the medical school.

120. William A. Bennett, interview with Marybeth Gasman, May 19, 2009.

121. William A. Bennett, interview with Marybeth Gasman, May 19, 2009. According

to Bennett, Hugh Gloster was so impressed with his work and dedication that he asked Bennett to leave his job with the federal government and come to Morehouse as the dean of the Medical Education Program. Bennett declined the offer, worried that the doctors in the medical program would not look highly upon his PhD, preferring instead a dean with an MD.

122. Louis W. Sullivan, interview for Morehouse School of Medicine Public Relations Department, 2007, Public Relations Department, Morehouse School of Medicine.

123. Louis W. Sullivan, interview for Morehouse School of Medicine Public Relations Department, 2007, Public Relations Department, Morehouse School of Medicine.

124. Steven Muller, "Higher Education or Higher Skilling?" *Daedalus*, vol. 103, no. 4 (Fall 1974), 148–158.

125. Jimmy Carter, interview with Marybeth Gasman, Sept. 28, 2008; Louis W. Sullivan, interview with Marybeth Gasman, Jan. 11, 2008.

126. Jimmy Carter, interview with Marybeth Gasman, Sept. 28, 2008.

127. Rhodes Haverty, interview with Marybeth Gasman, Feb. 11, 2009.

128. Louis W. Sullivan, interview with Marybeth Gasman, Jan. 11, 2008. William A. Bennett also mentioned this during his interview with Marybeth Gasman, May 19, 2009.

129. Rhodes Haverty, interview with Marybeth Gasman, Feb. 11, 2009; William A. Bennett also mentioned this during his interview with Marybeth Gasman, May 19, 2009.

130. William A. Bennett, interview with Marybeth Gasman, May 19, 2009.

131. Louis W. Sullivan, interview for Morehouse School of Medicine Public Relations Department, 2007, Public Relations Department, Morehouse School of Medicine.

132. Louis W. Sullivan, interview for Morehouse School of Medicine Public Relations Department, 2007, Public Relations Department, Morehouse School of Medicine.

133. Louis W. Sullivan, interview for Morehouse School of Medicine Public Relations Department, 2007, Public Relations Department, Morehouse School of Medicine; Yvonne Gloster, interview with Marybeth Gasman, Feb. 10, 2008; Ginger Sullivan, interview with Marybeth Gasman, Oct. 8, 2008. Bill Bennett also recalls this depiction of the New York meeting. See William A. Bennett, interview with Marybeth Gasman, May 19, 2009.

134. Ginger Sullivan, interview with Marybeth Gasman, Oct. 8, 2008.

135. Louis W. Sullivan, interview for Morehouse School of Medicine Public Relations Department 2007, Public Relations Department, Morehouse School of Medicine.

136. Ginger Sullivan, interview with Marybeth Gasman, Oct. 8, 2008.

137. James Story, interview with Marybeth Gasman, Mar. 24, 2008.

138. Ginger Sullivan, interview with Marybeth Gasman, Oct. 8, 2008.

139. Ginger Sullivan, interview with Marybeth Gasman, Oct. 8, 2008. Additional information gleaned from Louis W. Sullivan's curriculum vitae and the oral history interviews completed for this book.

140. William A. Bennett, interview with Marybeth Gasman, May 19, 2009.

Chapter 3 · *Building His Bike as He Rides It*

1. "Louis W. Sullivan Appointed Dean of Medical Education Program," press release, April 4, 1975, Morehouse School of Medicine Archives, Atlanta, Georgia.

2. Arnold Fleischman and Carol Pierannuzi, *Politics in Georgia* (Athens: University of Georgia Press, 2007).

3. Clarence Stone, *Regime Politics: Governing Atlanta, 1946–1988* (Lawrence: University Press of Kansas, 1989); Fleischman and Pierannuzi, *Politics in Georgia*.

4. Louis W. Sullivan, interview for Morehouse School of Medicine Public Relations Department, 2007, in the possession of the Public Relations Department, Morehouse School of Medicine, Atlanta, Georgia.

5. *New Georgia Encyclopedia* website, www.georgiaencyclopedia.org, accessed Jan. 25, 2010.

6. Ibid.

7. Louis W. Sullivan, interview for Morehouse School of Medicine, Public Relations Department, 2007, Public Relations Department, Morehouse School of Medicine.

8. "Louis W. Sullivan Appointed Dean," press release.

9. Louis W. Sullivan, interview for Morehouse School of Medicine, Public Relations Department, 2007, Public Relations Department, Morehouse School of Medicine.

10. Louis W. Sullivan, interview for Morehouse School of Medicine, Public Relations Department, 2007, Public Relations Department, Morehouse School of Medicine.

11. For an overview of the starving of Black colleges, see Marybeth Gasman, *Envisioning Black Colleges: A History of the United Negro College Fund* (Baltimore: Johns Hopkins University Press, 2009); Henry Drewry and Humphrey Doermann, *Stand and Prosper: Private Black Colleges and Universities* (Princeton, NJ: Princeton University Press, 1999).

12. Louis W. Sullivan, interview for Morehouse School of Medicine, Public Relations Department, 2007, Public Relations Department, Morehouse School of Medicine.

13. Gary MaGaha, interview with Marybeth Gasman, Mar. 12, 2007.

14. David Satcher, interview with Marybeth Gasman, Apr. 7, 2009.

15. Charles Stephens, interview with Marybeth Gasman, Apr. 7, 2008.

16. Asa G. Yancey Sr., interview with Marybeth Gasman, May 13, 2008.

17. Gary MaGaha, interview with Marybeth Gasman, Mar. 12, 2007.

18. Angela Franklin, interview with Marybeth Gasman, June 14, 2008.

19. Angela Franklin, interview with Marybeth Gasman, June 14, 2008.

20. Marjorie Smith, interview with Marybeth Gasman, Feb. 25, 2008.

21. Marjorie Smith, interview with Marybeth Gasman, Feb. 25, 2008; David Mann, interview with Marybeth Gasman, Feb. 26, 2009; James Story, interview with Marybeth Gasman, Mar. 24, 2008.

22. Sarah Austin, interview with Marybeth Gasman, June 6, 2008; Louis W. Sullivan, interview with Marybeth Gasman, Feb. 25, 2009.

23. Louis W. Sullivan, interview with Marybeth Gasman, Feb. 25, 2009.

24. Louis W. Sullivan, interview for Morehouse School of Medicine, Public Relations Department, 2007, Public Relations Department, Morehouse School of Medicine.

25. Drewry and Doermann, *Stand and Prosper*.

26. Louis W. Sullivan, interview for Morehouse School of Medicine, Public Relations Department, 2007, Public Relations Department, Morehouse School of Medicine; Yvonne Gloster, interview with Marybeth Gasman, Feb. 10, 2008.

27. Louis W. Sullivan, interview for Morehouse School of Medicine, Public Relations Department, 2007, Public Relations Department, Morehouse School of Medicine.

28. Charles Stephens, interview with Marybeth Gasman, Apr. 7, 2008.

29. Information on the funding of these faculty positions is in the Morehouse College folders, 1975–1980, Rockefeller Archive Center, Sleepy Hollow, New York.

30. Louis W. Sullivan, interview with Marybeth Gasman, Jan. 11, 2008.

31. Louis W. Sullivan, interview with Marybeth Gasman, Jan. 11, 2008. See also Marjorie Smith, interview with Marybeth Gasman, Feb. 25, 2008; James Story, interview with Marybeth Gasman, Mar. 24, 2008; David Mann, interview with Marybeth Gasman, Feb. 26, 2009.

32. Louis W. Sullivan, interview with Marybeth Gasman, Jan. 11, 2008; Marjorie Smith, interview with Marybeth Gasman, Feb. 25, 2008; James Story, interview with Marybeth Gasman, Mar. 24, 2008.

33. David Mann, interview with Marybeth Gasman, Feb. 26, 2009.

34. Louis W. Sullivan, interview with Marybeth Gasman, Jan. 11, 2008; David Mann, interview with Marybeth Gasman, Feb. 26, 2009.

35. Louis W. Sullivan, interview with Marybeth Gasman, Jan. 11, 2008; David Mann, interview with Marybeth Gasman, Feb. 26, 2009. James Story also recounted this incident in his interview with Marybeth Gasman, Mar. 24, 2008.

36. "SMMC: The Development of a Dream," *Tablet* (Morehouse School of Medicine), vol. 5, no. 3 (Fall 1980), 5. Available at the HBCU [Historically Black Colleges and Universities] Library Alliance's Digital Collection website, http://contentdm.auctr.edu/.

37. Delutha King, interview with Marybeth Gasman, June 10, 2008.

38. "SMMC: The Development of a Dream."

39. David Mann, interview with Marybeth Gasman, Feb. 26, 2009; Similar recollections were also made by Marjorie Smith, interview with Marybeth Gasman, Feb. 25, 2008; James Story, interview with Marybeth Gasman, Mar. 24, 2008.

40. David Mann, interview with Marybeth Gasman, Feb. 26, 2009.

41. Larry Cuban, *How Scholars Trumped Teachers: Change without Reform in University Curriculum, Teaching, and Research, 1890–1990* (New York: Teachers College Press, 1999).

42. Louis W. Sullivan, interview with Marybeth Gasman, Jan. 11, 2008.

43. "New Name Adopted," *Tablet* (Morehouse School of Medicine), vol. 1, no. 3 (Fall 1976), 1.

44. Office of the Administrator, Health Resources Administration, U.S. Department of Health, Education, and Welfare, "Graduate Medical Education: An Overview of Societal Concern, Social Policy, and Historical Developments; A Background Paper Prepared for the Graduate Medical Education National Advisory Committee," March 1977.

45. Institute of Medicine, Division of Health Sciences Policy, *Medical Education and Societal Needs: A Planning Report for the Health Professions* (Washington, DC: National Academy Press, July 1983).

46. Louis W. Sullivan, "Our Institutional Mission," Dean Notes, *Tablet* (Morehouse School of Medicine), vol. 2, no. 1 (Spring 1977), 2.

47. Cuban, *How Scholars Trumped Teachers*, 180.

48. For comparison data, see Paul Starr, *The Social Transformation of American Medicine: The Rise of a Sovereign Profession and the Making of a Vast Industry* (New York: Basic Books, 1982). The Liaison Committee on Medical Education is sponsored by the Association of American Medical Colleges and the American Medical Association.

49. Charles Stephens, interview with Marybeth Gasman, Apr. 7, 2008; Shirley Desaussure, interview with Marybeth Gasman, Oct. 11, 2007.

50. Charles Stephens, interview with Marybeth Gasman, Apr. 7, 2008. This observation was reiterated by Shirley Desaussure, interview with Marybeth Gasman, Oct. 11, 2007.

51. This statement is based on a thorough review of all medical schools in the United States. Although Dartmouth is a college in name, it is much larger and has graduate programs.

52. Charles Stephens, interview with Marybeth Gasman, Apr. 7, 2008; Shirley Desaussure, interview with Marybeth Gasman, Oct. 11, 2007.

53. Christopher Jencks and David Riesman, *The Academic Revolution* (Chicago: University of Chicago Press, 1968), 217.

54. The Liaison Committee on Medical Education (LCME) comprises representatives from the American Medical Association (AMA) and the American Association of Medical Colleges (AAMC). The executive secretariat moves every two years from the AMA to the AAMC and back. Each organization has a full-time executive secretary for the LCME. As a result of the 1973 LCME ruling, the following two-year schools became four-year, MD degree–granting institutions: University of Nevada, Las Vegas; University of North Dakota; University of South Dakota; Dartmouth College; and Morehouse School of Medicine. For procedural information and a history of LCME actions, see www.lcme.org.

55. Louis W. Sullivan, interview with Marybeth Gasman, Jan. 11, 2008.

56. Louis W. Sullivan, interview with Marybeth Gasman, Mar. 13, 2009.

57. Louis W. Sullivan, interview with Marybeth Gasman, Apr. 14, 2010.

58. "SMMC Gets $1 Million State Grant," *Tablet* (Morehouse School of Medicine), vol. 2, no. 1 (Spring 1977), 1.

59. Ibid.

60. Louis W. Sullivan, interview with Marybeth Gasman, Jan. 11, 2008; Jimmy Carter, interview with Marybeth Gasman, Sept. 28, 2008.

61. "Federal Appropriations to Howard University," www.whitehouse.gov, accessed June 6, 2009; "Federal Appropriations to Gallaudet University," www.whitehouse.gov, accessed June 6, 2009.

62. Louis W. Sullivan, interview with Marybeth Gasman, Jan. 11, 2008; Jimmy Carter, interview with Marybeth Gasman, Sept. 28, 2008.

63. Jimmy Carter, interview with Marybeth Gasman, Sept. 28, 2008.

64. "Federal Appropriations to Howard University."

65. "Federal Appropriations to Gallaudet University."

66. For a thorough discussion of the Carter administration's initiatives related to health care and medicine, see Starr, *Social Transformation of American Medicine.*

67. Jimmy Carter, interview with Marybeth Gasman, Sept. 28, 2008.

68. Jimmy Carter, interview with Marybeth Gasman, Sept. 28, 2008.

69. Louis W. Sullivan, interview with Marybeth Gasman, Jan. 11, 2008.

70. Andrew Young, interview with Marybeth Gasman, June 8, 2008.

71. Andrew Young, interview with Marybeth Gasman, June 8, 2008.

72. Charles Stephens, interview with Marybeth Gasman, Apr. 7, 2008. This was corroborated by Sarah Austin, interview with Marybeth Gasman, June 10, 2008.

73. Charles Stephens, interview with Marybeth Gasman, Apr. 7, 2008.

74. Charles Stephens, interview with Marybeth Gasman, Apr. 7, 2008. This story was also reiterated by Louis W. Sullivan, interview with Marybeth Gasman, Feb. 18, 2008.

75. Louis W. Sullivan, interview with Marybeth Gasman, Feb. 18, 2008.

76. See Christopher Jencks and David Riesman, "The American Negro College," *Harvard Educational Review*, vol. 37, no. 1 (Winter 1967), 3–60. For an analysis of the impact of the article, see Marybeth Gasman, "Salvaging 'Academic Disaster Areas': The Black College Response to Christopher Jencks' and David Riesman's 1967 *Harvard Educational Review* Article," *Journal of Higher Education*, vol. 77, no. 2 (2006), 317–352.

77. Jencks and Riesman, "American Negro College"; Gasman, "Salvaging 'Academic Disaster Areas.'" For a full discussion of Gloster's role, see Gasman, *Envisioning Black Colleges*.

78. Yvonne Gloster, interview with Marybeth Gasman, Feb. 10, 2008.

79. Yvonne Gloster, interview with Marybeth Gasman, Feb. 10, 2008.

80. Louis W. Sullivan, interview with Marybeth Gasman, Jan. 11, 2008; Charles Stephens, interview with Marybeth Gasman, Apr. 7, 2008.

81. Louis W. Sullivan, interview with Marybeth Gasman, Jan. 11, 2008.

82. Louis W. Sullivan, interview with Marybeth Gasman, Jan. 11, 2008; Charles Stephens, interview with Marybeth Gasman, Apr. 7, 2008.

83. Clinton Warner, interview with Marybeth Gasman, Feb. 10, 2008.

84. "Morehouse Begins New Era," *Atlanta Constitution*, Sept. 11, 1978, 1A.

85. James D. Anderson, *The Education of Blacks in the South, 1865–1930* (Chapel Hill: University of North Carolina Press, 1988).

86. Louis W. Sullivan, interview with Marybeth Gasman, Feb. 18, 2008.

87. Andrew Young, interview with Marybeth Gasman, June 8, 2008.

88. Andrew Young, interview with Marybeth Gasman, June 8, 2008.

89. Ginger Sullivan, interview with Marybeth Gasman, Oct. 8, 2008; Friends of Morehouse School of Medicine file, Morehouse School of Medicine Archives.

90. For more information on capitation programs, see the corresponding folder, Morehouse School of Medicine Archives.

91. "Pfizer's Curti Named to Morehouse School of Medicine Board," press release, Aug. 31, 1987, Morehouse School of Medicine Archives.

92. James Story, interview with Marybeth Gasman, Mar. 24, 2008.

93. James Story, interview with Marybeth Gasman, Mar. 24, 2008. See also the files on the first medical school class, Morehouse School of Medicine Archives.

94. Louis W. Sullivan, interview with Marybeth Gasman, Jan. 11, 2008.

95. David Mann, interview with Marybeth Gasman, Feb. 28, 2009. See also the file regarding a vote of no confidence in the dean, which includes the corresponding board minutes, Morehouse School of Medicine Archive.

96. David Mann, interview with Marybeth Gasman, Feb. 28, 2009.

97. Louis W. Sullivan, interview with Marybeth Gasman, Mar. 15, 2009.

98. David Mann, interview with Marybeth Gasman, Feb. 28, 2009; Louis W. Sullivan, interview with Marybeth Gasman, Mar. 15, 2009.

99. Louis W. Sullivan, interview with Marybeth Gasman, Mar. 15, 2009; Edward Allen Jones, *A Candle in the Dark: A History of Morehouse College* (Atlanta: Judson Press, 1967).

100. Yvonne Gloster, interview with Marybeth Gasman, Feb. 10, 2008. See the Hugh

Gloster papers, Morehouse College Archives, for ample evidence of his relationship with local media.

101. See the file folder on Board of Trustee meeting minutes from 1978 for details on the "no confidence" meeting, Morehouse School of Medicine Archives.

102. Louis W. Sullivan, interview with Marybeth Gasman, Mar. 15, 2009.

103. Charles V. Willie and Ronald R. Edmonds, eds., *Black Colleges in America: Challenge, Development, Survival* (New York: Teachers College Press, 1978); Joy A. Williamson, *Radicalizing the Ebony Tower: Black Colleges and the Black Freedom Struggle in Mississippi* (New York: Teachers College Press, 2008).

104. Williamson, *Radicalizing the Ebony Tower;* Marybeth Gasman, "Perceptions of Black College Presidents: Sorting Through Stereotypes and Reality to Gain a Complex Picture," *American Education Research Journal* (forthcoming, 2011).

105. Transfer articulation agreements are in the Morehouse School of Medicine Archives.

106. Morehouse School of Medicine, "A Short History," unpublished manuscript, May 4, 1988.

107. "Charter Class Completes Studies at SMMC," *Tablet* (Morehouse School of Medicine), vol. 5, no. 2 (Summer 1980), 1.

Chapter 4 · Coming into Its Own

1. Articles of incorporation of the Morehouse School of Medicine Inc., Morehouse School of Medicine Archives, Atlanta, Georgia.

2. James Story, interview with Marybeth Gasman, Mar. 24, 2008.

3. Louis W. Sullivan, interview with Marybeth Gasman, Jan. 11, 2008.

4. Louis W. Sullivan, interview with Marybeth Gasman, Jan. 11, 2008.

5. Christopher Jencks and David Riesman, *The Academic Revolution* (Chicago: University of Chicago Press, 1968), 213.

6. See, for example, Jencks and Riesman, *Academic Revolution;* Paul Starr, *The Social Transformation of American Medicine: The Rise of a Sovereign Profession and the Making of a Vast Industry* (New York: Basic Books, 1982).

7. Louis W. Sullivan, interview with Marybeth Gasman, Jan. 11, 2008.

8. "Groundbreaking Ceremonies at Morehouse," *Lovely Atlanta,* Fall 1980, 12–13. See also "Groundbreaking Ceremonies Set for Morehouse Medical School Building," *Informer,* 1980, 16. Both articles are in the Morehouse School of Medicine Archives.

9. Vida L. Avery, "A Fateful Hour in Black Higher Education: The Creation of the Atlanta University System," PhD diss., Georgia State University, 2003.

10. Louis W. Sullivan, interview with Marybeth Gasman, Jan. 11, 2008.

11. "Transition Campaign Committee Highly Successful," *Tablet* (Morehouse School of Medicine), vol. 1, no. 4 (Summer 1982), 3. Available at the HBCU [Historically Black Colleges and Universities] Library Alliance's Digital Collection website, http://contentdm .auctr.edu/.

12. Louis W. Sullivan, interview with Marybeth Gasman, Mar. 11, 2008.

13. Louis W. Sullivan, interview with Marybeth Gasman, Mar. 11, 2008.

14. "Vice President at Morehouse," *Atlanta Constitution,* July 22, 1982.

15. Spencer Rich, "Tax Cuts Aid Minorities Least, Rights Unit Says," *Washington Post*, May 5, 1981; Spencer Rich, "Big-City Mayors See Reagan Budget Toll in Layoffs and Cuts," *Washington Post*, May 2, 1981.

16. Louis W. Sullivan, interview with Marybeth Gasman, Jan. 11, 2008. Eventually, the U.S. Supreme Court ruled against Bob Jones University and President Reagan, rescinding the institution's tax-exempt status unless the institution rid itself of its segregated past. See *Bob Jones University v. United States*, 461 U.S. 574 (1983). See also Mark Shields, "Singing the Bob Jones School Song," *Washington Post*, May 27, 1983; Caroline R. Herron and Michael Wright, "Reagan Takes the Blame and the Heat as Well," *New York Times*, Jan. 24, 1982; Walter Shapiro and Diane Camper, "Reagan's Civil-Rights Woes," *Newsweek*, June 6, 1983.

17. Louis W. Sullivan, interview with Marybeth Gasman, Jan. 11, 2008.

18. "Morehouse Medical Comes of Age," *Ebony*, November 1982, 74–78. See also "Vice President Bush Announces $2.6 Million Challenge Grant," *Tablet* (Morehouse School of Medicine), vol. 2, no. 1 (Fall 1982), 1, 3.

19. Louis W. Sullivan, interview for Morehouse School of Medicine Public Relations Department, 2007, in the possession of the Public Relations Department, Morehouse School of Medicine, Atlanta, Georgia.

20. Louis W. Sullivan, interview with Marybeth Gasman, Jan. 11, 2008.

21. Louis W. Sullivan, "Dean Notes," *Tablet* (Morehouse School of Medicine), vol. 2, no. 2 (Winter 1983), 2.

22. Charles Seabrook, "Morehouse Dean Gains International Influence," *Atlanta Constitution*, May 23, 1982.

23. Ibid.

24. Charles Stephens, interview with Marybeth Gasman, Apr. 7, 2008.

25. David Rogers, *American Medicine: Challenges for the 1980s* (Cambridge, MA: Ballinger, 1978); J. R. Schofield, *New and Expanded Medical Schools, Mid-Century to the 1980s: An Analysis of Changes and Recommendations for Improving the Education of Physicians* (San Francisco: Jossey-Bass, 1984). A scan of *Time, Newsweek*, and *U.S. News and World Report* magazines makes these factors evident.

26. Charles Hatcher, interview with Marybeth Gasman, July 23, 2009.

27. Charles Hatcher, interview with Marybeth Gasman, July 23, 2009. See also Emory University files, Morehouse School of Medicine Archives.

28. Charles Hatcher, interview with Marybeth Gasman, July 23, 2009.

29. Charles Hatcher, interview with Marybeth Gasman, July 23, 2009.

30. "Morehouse Begins New Era," *Atlanta Constitution*, Sept. 11, 1978, 1A.

31. Dartmouth College started out as a four-year program in 1797, but Abraham Flexner, in his 1910 report on medical education, deemed it too remote for clinical training. The last class to receive MDs from Dartmouth was that of 1914; subsequent students took their first two years of medical school at the New Hampshire institution and transferred elsewhere for their clinical years. This was the case until 1970; a new class of MDs graduated in 1974. The University of Mississippi also began as a two-year medical program on the flagship campus in Oxford, Mississippi, in 1903. The medical school was eventually moved to the state capital of Jackson, and the curriculum was expanded to four years. Lastly, the University of North Carolina opened its medical school in 1879, experiencing

164 Notes to Pages 78–84

an occasional closing during the early years. This institution, like its Mississippi counterpart, did not fare well in Abraham Flexner's report; it could not afford to upgrade the preclinical and clinical departments to meet Flexner's guidelines and subsequently closed. Eventually the institution reopened, with the help of some dedicated faculty members, offering a two-year program with transfer agreements to medical schools in the Northeast and South. With the help of a General Assembly appropriation for a medial hospital in 1947, the University of North Carolina graduated its first class of MDs in 1954. See Carlton Chapman, *Dartmouth Medical School: The First 176 Years* (Hanover, NH: University Press of New England, 1973); "History" and "Mission," the University of Mississippi Medical Center website, www.umc.edu/medical_center/overview.html; David G. Sansing, *The University of Mississippi: A Sesquicentennial History* (Oxford: University of Mississippi Press, 1999); "History," the University of North Carolina Medical School website, www.med.unc.edu/www/about/history/; William D. Snider, *Light on the Hill: A History of the University of North Carolina at Chapel Hill* (Chapel Hill: University of North Carolina Press, 1992).

32. "AMA Official 'Highly Impressed' by Morehouse Visit," *Tablet* (Morehouse School of Medicine), vol. 1, no. 2 (Winter 1981/1982), 1. See also Rogers, *American Medicine*; Schofield, *New and Expanded Medical Schools*.

33. "AMA Official 'Highly Impressed'."

34. Ibid.

35. Institute of Health, Division of Health Sciences Policy, *Medical Education and Societal Needs: A Planning Report for the Health Professions* (Washington, DC: National Academy Press, July 1983).

36. "Louis W. Sullivan Inaugurated as First President," *Tablet* (Morehouse School of Medicine), vol. 2, no. 1 (Spring 1983), 1.

37. Charles Hatcher, interview with Marybeth Gasman, July 23, 2008; Jonas Shulman, interview with Marybeth Gasman, May 13, 2008.

38. Jonas Shulman, interview with Marybeth Gasman, May 13, 2008. See also Rogers, *American Medicine*; Schofield, *New and Expanded Medical Schools*.

39. Charles Hatcher, interview with Marybeth Gasman, July 23, 2008.

40. Charles Hatcher, interview with Marybeth Gasman, July 23, 2008.

41. Asa G. Yancey Sr., interview with Marybeth Gasman, May 13, 2008.

42. Charles Hatcher, interview with Marybeth Gasman, July 23, 2008. This story is also recounted by Louis W. Sullivan, interview with Marybeth Gasman, Jan. 11, 2008.

43. Charles Hatcher, interview with Marybeth Gasman, July 23, 2008.

44. Clinton Warner, interview with Marybeth Gasman, Feb. 10, 2008.

45. Louis W. Sullivan, interview with Marybeth Gasman, Jan. 11, 2008; Gary MaGaha, interview with Marybeth Gasman, Feb. 26, 2009.

46. Charles Hatcher, interview with Marybeth Gasman, July 23, 2009. See also Emory University files, Morehouse School of Medicine Archives.

47. Charles Hatcher, interview with Marybeth Gasman, July 23, 2009. See also Emory University files, Morehouse School of Medicine Archives.

48. Gary MaGaha, interview with Marybeth Gasman, February 26, 2009.

49. See the Liaison Committee on Medical Education file, Morehouse School of Medicine Archives.

50. "First 21 Morehouse Medical Grads Get Bonus—School's Accreditation," *Atlanta Constitution*, May 2, 1985, 30A.

51. Ibid.

52. Ibid.

53. "Atlanta-Based Foundation Benefits Morehouse School of Medicine," press release, Aug. 12, 1987, Morehouse School of Medicine Archives, Atlanta, Georgia.

54. Morehouse School of Medicine, "A Short History," unpublished manuscript, May 4, 1988. For details on the doctor surplus, see Institute of Medicine, *Medical Education*.

55. Walter Sullivan to C. A. Scott at the *Atlanta Daily World*, Oct. 15, 1987, Morehouse School of Medicine Archives.

56. "Tate Supports Morehouse Aid," *Atlanta Voice*, Mar. 21, 1987.

57. Joe Frank Harris, interview with Marybeth Gasman, July 17, 2008.

58. Jasper Dorsey, "Georgia Needs Commitment of Higher Education," *Athens Metropolitan Area News*, May 1, 1989.

59. "Robert W. Johnson Foundation Aids Morehouse School of Medicine Clinical Development," *Atlanta World*, Aug. 25, 1987.

60. Institute of Medicine, *Medical Education*.

61. Barbara Bush, interview with Marybeth Gasman, Mar. 26, 2009.

62. Barbara Bush, interview with Marybeth Gasman, Mar. 26, 2009.

63. "Dave Winfield of New York Yankees Elected to Morehouse School of Medicine Board," press release, May 5, 1987, Morehouse School of Medicine Archives.

64. "Dave Winfield Named to Morehouse Medial School Board," *Los Angles Firestone Park News*, June 18, 1987.

65. Margaret Carlson, "Barbara Bush: Down-to-Earth First Lady," *Time*, Jan. 23, 1989.

66. Barbara Bush, interview with Marybeth Gasman, Mar. 26, 2009. Barbara Bush's estimation was confirmed with Carrie Dumas, the director of alumni at Morehouse School of Medicine.

67. Barbara Bush, interview with Marybeth Gasman, Mar. 26, 2009.

68. Barbara Bush, interview with Marybeth Gasman, Mar. 26, 2009. This thought was reiterated by George H. W. Bush, interview with Marybeth Gasman, Mar. 26, 2009.

69. George H. W. Bush, interview with Marybeth Gasman, Mar. 26, 2009.

70. Louis W. Sullivan, interview with Marybeth Gasman, Mar. 7, 2008; Clinton Warner, interview with Marybeth Gasman, Feb. 10, 2008.

71. Louis W. Sullivan, interview for Morehouse School of Medicine Public Relations Department, 2007, Public Relations Department, Morehouse School of Medicine.

72. Louis W. Sullivan, interview for Morehouse School of Medicine Public Relations Department, 2007, Public Relations Department, Morehouse School of Medicine.

73. George H. W. Bush, interview with Marybeth Gasman, Mar. 26, 2009.

74. Chester A. Higgins Sr., "Dr. Sullivan Gets $250,000 Morehouse Pay; Medical School Names New President," *Augusta Focus*, Apr. 26, 1989; "Sullivan Gets Morehouse Pay After All," *Brooklyn Big Red News*, Apr. 8, 1989.

75. Clinton Warner learned that Boeing gave bonuses to its employees who went to work for the White House and that, as a result, Boeing was accused of buying their loyalty. He thought that Morehouse would be similarly accused. See Chester A. Higgins Sr., "Sul-

livan to Get Sabbatical Pay," *Portland Skanner*, Apr. 5, 1989; Clinton Warner, interview with Marybeth Gasman, Feb. 10, 2008.

76. Louis W. Sullivan, interview with Marybeth Gasman, Mar. 7, 2008; Clinton Warner, interview with Marybeth Gasman, Feb. 10, 2008.

Chapter 5 · Leadership in Transition

1. "New Morehouse Med School Chief Appointed," *San Francisco Sun Reporter*, May 3, 1989; "Goodman Named President of Morehouse School of Medicine," *Los Angeles Firestone Park News*, Apr. 27, 1989; "Dr. James A. Goodman Named Morehouse Med School Prexy," *Jet*, Apr. 10, 1989.

2. James Goodman, interview with Marybeth Gasman, Apr. 20, 2009.

3. Paul Starr, *The Social Transformation of American Medicine: The Rise of a Sovereign Profession and the Making of a Vast Industry* (New York: Basic Books, 1982).

4. James Goodman, interview with Marybeth Gasman, Apr. 20, 2009.

5. James Goodman, interview with Marybeth Gasman, Apr. 20, 2009.

6. Cynthia Durcanin, "Insider Tapped as President of Morehouse Medical School," *Atlanta Constitution*, Mar. 11, 1989, 1C.

7. Ibid.

8. James Goodman, interview with Marybeth Gasman, Apr. 20, 2009.

9. Louis W. Sullivan, interview with Marybeth Gasman, Feb. 27, 2009.

10. Louis W. Sullivan, interview with Marybeth Gasman, Feb. 27, 2009. This sentiment was reiterated by Gary MaGaha, interview with Marybeth Gasman, Feb. 26, 2008.

11. James Goodman, interview with Marybeth Gasman, Apr. 20, 2009. See also Angela Franklin, interview with Marybeth Gasman, June 14, 2008.

12. Gary MaGaha, interview with Marybeth Gasman, Feb. 26, 2009.

13. James Goodman, interview with Marybeth Gasman, Apr. 20, 2009.

14. Gary MaGaha, interview with Marybeth Gasman, Feb. 26, 2008; Angela Franklin, interview with Marybeth Gasman, June 14, 2008.

15. James Goodman, interview with Marybeth Gasman, Apr. 20, 2009.

16. James Goodman, interview with Marybeth Gasman, Apr. 20, 2009.

17. James D. Anderson, *The Education of Blacks in the South, 1865–1930* (Chapel Hill: University of North Carolina Press, 1988).

18. Ibid. See also W. E. B. DuBois, *Black Reconstruction in America* (New York: Oxford University Press, 2007).

19. James Goodman, interview with Marybeth Gasman, Apr. 20, 2009.

20. James Goodman, interview with Marybeth Gasman, Apr. 20, 2009.

21. See the correspondence file for James Goodman, Morehouse School of Medicine Archives, Atlanta, Georgia.

22. James Goodman, interview with Marybeth Gasman, Apr. 20, 2009. See also the correspondence file for James Goodman, Morehouse School of Medicine Archives.

23. James Goodman, interview with Marybeth Gasman, Apr. 20, 2009.

24. James Goodman, interview with Marybeth Gasman, Apr. 20, 2009. For more in-

formation on the accomplishments of James Goodman while president, see the Morehouse School of Medicine Archives.

25. Bernadette Burden, "400 Students Take Part in Conference on Sex, Drugs, and Nutrition," *Atlanta Constitution*, Mar. 5, 1989.

26. *Morehouse School of Medicine National Alumni News*, vol. 1, no. 3 (May 1993).

27. James Goodman, interview with Marybeth Gasman, Apr. 20, 2009. See also Morehouse School of Medicine Board of Trustees minutes, 1992, Morehouse School of Medicine Archives.

28. James Goodman, interview with Marybeth Gasman, Apr. 20, 2009. See also Morehouse School of Medicine Board of Trustees minutes, 1992, Morehouse School of Medicine Archives.

29. James Goodman, interview with Marybeth Gasman, April 20, 2009.

30. Marybeth Gasman, Benjamin Baez, Noah Drezner, Katherine Sedgwick, and Christopher Tudico, "Historically Black Colleges and Universities: Recent Trends," *Academe* (Jan.–Feb. 2007), 69–77.

31. See the Morehouse School of Medicine Board of Trustees minutes, 1992–1993, Morehouse School of Medicine Archives.

32. Walter Sullivan, interview with Marybeth Gasman, July 23, 2008.

33. Louis W. Sullivan, interview with Marybeth Gasman, Feb. 14, 2009.

34. Louis W. Sullivan, interview with Marybeth Gasman, Feb. 14, 2009.

35. Gayle Converse, interview with Marybeth Gasman, Apr. 10, 2008.

36. Ginger Sullivan, interview with Marybeth Gasman, Oct. 8, 2008.

37. For information on the everyday happenings at the institution, see the *Tablet* between 1989–2002, available at the HBCU [Historically Black Colleges and Universities] Library Alliance's Digital Collection website, http://contentdm.auctr.edu/.

Chapter 6 · A Controversy Erupts

1. James Gavin, interview with Marybeth Gasman, Aug. 14, 2009. See also James Gavin's professional biography, Morehouse School of Medicine Archives, Atlanta, Georgia.

2. James Gavin, interview with Marybeth Gasman, Aug. 14, 2009; Blakely correspondence, Morehouse School of Medicine Archives.

3. James Gavin, interview with Marybeth Gasman, Aug. 14, 2009.

4. Louis W. Sullivan, interview with Marybeth Gasman, Feb. 14, 2009; Blakely correspondence, Morehouse School of Medicine Archives.

5. Louis W. Sullivan, interview with Marybeth Gasman, Jan. 11, 2008.

6. Louis W. Sullivan, interview with Marybeth Gasman, Feb. 14, 2009.

7. James Gavin, interview with Marybeth Gasman, Aug. 14, 2009; Blakely correspondence, Morehouse School of Medicine Archives.

8. James Gavin, interview with Marybeth Gasman, Aug. 14, 2009; Blakely correspondence, Morehouse School of Medicine Archives.

9. James Gavin, interview with Marybeth Gasman, Aug. 14, 2009.

10. James Gavin, interview with Marybeth Gasman, Aug. 14, 2009.

11. Louis W. Sullivan, interview with Marybeth Gasman, Feb. 14, 2009.

12. Louis W. Sullivan, interview with Marybeth Gasman, Jan. 11, 2008.

13. This recollection was by Louis W. Sullivan, interview with Marybeth Gasman, Jan. 11, 2008. See also James Gavin, interview with Marybeth Gasman, Aug. 14, 2009.

14. Michael D. Cohen, *Leadership and Ambiguity: The American College President* (Cambridge, MA: Harvard Business Press, 1986); Laurence W. Weill, *Out in Front: The College President as the Face of the Institution* (Washington, DC: American Council on Education, 2009).

15. Sonny Lufrano, "Building Morehouse School of Medicine's Brand," *Atlanta Business Chronicle* (July 25–31, 2003), 12.

16. James Gavin, interview with Marybeth Gasman, Aug. 14, 2009.

17. James Gavin, interview with Marybeth Gasman, Aug. 14, 2009. Given the school's very strong ties to Washington, D.C., which are supported by myriad primary sources in the Morehouse School of Medicine Archives, Gavin could have had a point. Nonetheless, the medical school was a product of interracial cooperation in the city of Atlanta and state of Georgia.

18. James Gavin, interview with Marybeth Gasman, Aug. 14, 2009.

19. James Gavin, interview with Marybeth Gasman, Aug. 14, 2009. The *Tablet* (Morehouse School of Medicine) details the specific actions of Gavin during this time. Issues of the *Tablet* are available at the HBCU [Historically Black Colleges and Universities] Library Alliance's Digital Collection website, http://contentdm.auctr.edu/.

20. James Gavin, interview with Marybeth Gasman, Aug. 14, 2009.

21. Lufrano, "Building."

22. Ibid.

23. The dearth of research assistants and graduate programs is captured in interviews with Morehouse School of Medicine faculty and in the Morehouse School of Medicine Board of Trustee minutes during Gavin's presidency. See the Morehouse School of Medicine Archives.

24. James Gavin, interview with Marybeth Gasman, Aug. 14, 2009. See also the program review file in the Morehouse School of Medicine Archives.

25. James Gavin, interview with Marybeth Gasman, Aug. 14, 2009. See also the program review file in the Morehouse School of Medicine Archives.

26. James Gavin, interview with Marybeth Gasman, Aug. 14, 2009.

27. Cohen, *Leadership and Ambiguity*; Weill, *Out in Front*.

28. James Gavin, interview with Marybeth Gasman, Aug. 14, 2009.

29. Louis W. Sullivan, interview with Marybeth Gasman, Jan. 11, 2008.

30. James Gavin, interview with Marybeth Gasman, Aug. 14, 2009.

31. James Gavin, interview with Marybeth Gasman, Aug. 14, 2009; Clinton Warner, interview with Marybeth Gasman, Feb. 10, 2008.

32. James Gavin, interview with Marybeth Gasman, Aug. 14, 2009; Clinton Warner, interview with Marybeth Gasman, Feb. 10, 2008.

33. Cohen, *Leadership and Ambiguity*; Weill, *Out in Front*.

34. James Gavin, interview with Marybeth Gasman, Aug. 14, 2009; Blakely correspondence, Morehouse School of Medicine Archives.

35. James Gavin, interview with Marybeth Gasman, Aug. 14, 2009.

36. Louis W. Sullivan, interview with Marybeth Gasman, Jan. 11, 2008.

37. James Gavin, interview with Marybeth Gasman, Aug. 14, 2009.

38. Clinton Warner, interview with Marybeth Gasman, Feb. 10, 2008.

39. Clinton Warner, interview with Marybeth Gasman, Feb. 10, 2008.

40. Andrea Jones, "Morehouse Med School to Ax Chief," *Atlanta Journal-Constitution*, Dec. 18, 2004, A1.

41. David Satcher, interview with Marybeth Gasman, Apr. 7, 2009.

42. David Satcher, interview with Marybeth Gasman, Apr. 7, 2009.

43. Jones, "Morehouse Med School." See also the letter from senior faculty to the Morehouse School of Medicine Board of Trustees, Dec. 9, 2004, Morehouse School of Medicine Archives.

44. Jones, "Morehouse Med School." See also the letter from senior faculty to the Morehouse School of Medicine Board of Trustees, Dec. 9, 2004, Morehouse School of Medicine Archives.

45. Jones, "Morehouse Med School."

46. Ibid. See also the memo from community leaders to the Morehouse School of Medicine Board of Trustees, undated, Morehouse School of Medicine Archives.

47. James Gavin, interview with Marybeth Gasman, Aug. 14, 2009.

48. James Gavin, interview with Marybeth Gasman, Aug. 14, 2009.

49. James Gavin, interview with Marybeth Gasman, Aug. 14, 2009; Jones, "Morehouse Med School."

50. James Gavin, interview with Marybeth Gasman, Aug. 14, 2009.

51. David Satcher, interview with Marybeth Gasman, Apr. 7, 2009; James Gavin, interview with Marybeth Gasman, Aug. 14, 2009.

52. Cohen, *Leadership and Ambiguity*; Weill, *Out in Front*.

53. David Satcher, interview with Marybeth Gasman, Apr. 7, 2009. See also the Morehouse School of Medicine Board of Trustee minutes, Morehouse School of Medicine Archives.

Chapter 7 · *Recovering from Turmoil*

1. David Satcher, interview with Marybeth Gasman, Apr. 7, 2009; James Gavin, interview with Marybeth Gasman, Aug, 14, 2009.

2. David Satcher, interview with Marybeth Gasman, Apr. 7, 2009; James Gavin, interview with Marybeth Gasman, Aug, 14, 2009.

3. David Satcher, interview with Marybeth Gasman, Apr. 7, 2009.

4. David Satcher, interview with Marybeth Gasman, Apr. 7, 2009. See also the Morehouse School of Medicine Board of Trustee minutes, Morehouse School of Medicine Archives, Atlanta, Georgia.

5. David Satcher, interview with Marybeth Gasman, Apr. 7, 2009.

6. David Satcher, interview with Marybeth Gasman, Apr. 7, 2009.

7. See the accreditation file, Morehouse School of Medicine Archives.

8. David Satcher, interview with Marybeth Gasman, Apr. 7, 2009. See also the David Satcher presidential file, Morehouse School of Medicine Archives.

9. David Satcher, interview with Marybeth Gasman, Apr. 7, 2009. The Morehouse School of Medicine Board of Trustees minutes, Morehouse School of Medicine Archives, account for the tense situation with Louis W. Sullivan but do not offer any specifics.

10. David Satcher, interview with Marybeth Gasman, Apr. 7, 2009. See also the David Satcher presidential file, Morehouse School of Medicine Archives.

11. David Satcher, interview with Marybeth Gasman, Apr. 7, 2009; John E. Maupin Jr., interview with Marybeth Gasman, Apr. 10, 2009.

12. David Satcher, interview with Marybeth Gasman, Apr. 7, 2009. See also the David Satcher presidential file, Morehouse School of Medicine Archives.

13. David Satcher, interview with Marybeth Gasman, Apr. 7, 2009.

14. Angela Franklin, interview with Marybeth Gasman, June 14, 2008.

15. See issues of the *Tablet* (Morehouse School of Medicine) and the file of correspondence with the community during Gavin's presidency, Morehouse School of Medicine Archives. The *Tablet* is also available at the HBCU [Historically Black Colleges and Universities] Library Alliance's Digital Collection website, http://contentdm.auctr.edu/.

16. David Satcher, interview with Marybeth Gasman, Apr. 7, 2009; Mary Kay Murphy, interview with Marybeth Gasman, Apr. 7, 2009.

17. David Satcher, interview with Marybeth Gasman, Apr. 7, 2009; Mary Kay Murphy, interview with Marybeth Gasman, Apr. 7, 2009.

18. David Satcher, interview with Marybeth Gasman, Apr. 7, 2009.

19. Marybeth Gasman and Sibby Anderson-Thompkins, *Fund Raising from Black College Alumni: Successful Strategies for Supporting Alma Mater* (Washington, DC: Council for Advancement and Support of Education [CASE], 2003).

20. Andrea Walton and Marybeth Gasman, eds. *Philanthropy, Volunteerism, and Fundraising in Higher Education* (New York: Pearson, 2008).

21. David Satcher, interview with Marybeth Gasman, Apr. 7, 2009; Mary Kay Murphy, interview with Marybeth Gasman, Apr. 7, 2009.

22. Delutha King, interview with Marybeth Gasman, June 10, 2009.

23. Louis W. Sullivan, interview with Marybeth Gasman, Jan. 11, 2008.

24. John E. Maupin Jr., official biographical sketch, Morehouse School of Medicine website, www.msm.edu/HomePage.aspx, accessed Nov. 1, 2009.

25. "L.A. Native Named Exec Vice President School of Medicine," *Los Angeles Herald Dispatch*, Apr. 13, 1998; "Dr. John E. Maupin Has Been Named Executive Vice President of Morehouse School of Medicine," *Atlanta Constitution*, May 18, 1989; "Former NDA President Named Exec VP of Morehouse School of Medicine," *Atlanta Daily World*, Apr. 21, 1989.

26. John E. Maupin Jr., interview with Marybeth Gasman, Apr. 10, 2009; James Goodman, interview with Marybeth Gasman, Apr. 20, 2009; Louis W. Sullivan, interview with Marybeth Gasman, Feb. 13, 2009; Mary Kay Murphy, interview with Marybeth Gasman, Apr. 7, 2009.

27. John E. Maupin Jr., interview with Marybeth Gasman, Apr. 10, 2009; David Satcher, interview with Marybeth Gasman, Apr. 7, 2009.

28. John E. Maupin Jr., interview with Marybeth Gasman, Apr. 10, 2009; David Satcher, interview with Marybeth Gasman, Apr. 7, 2009.

29. John E. Maupin Jr., interview with Marybeth Gasman, Apr. 10, 2009; Louis W.

Sullivan, interview with Marybeth Gasman, Feb. 13, 2009; James Goodman, interview with Marybeth Gasman, Apr. 20, 2009.

30. John E. Maupin Jr., interview with Marybeth Gasman, Apr. 13, 2008; Mary Kay Murphy, interview with Marybeth Gasman, Apr. 7, 2009.

31. John E. Maupin Jr., interview with Marybeth Gasman, Apr. 10, 2009.

32. Michael D. Cohen, *Leadership and Ambiguity: The American College President* (Cambridge, MA: Harvard Business Press, 1986); Laurence W. Weill, *Out in Front: The College President as the Face of the Institution* (Washington, DC: American Council on Education, 2009).

33. John E. Maupin Jr., interview with Marybeth Gasman, Apr. 10, 2009; James Goodman, interview with Marybeth Gasman, Apr. 20, 2009.

34. John E. Maupin Jr., interview with Marybeth Gasman, Apr. 10, 2009; James Goodman, interview with Marybeth Gasman, Apr. 20, 2009.

35. See the Morehouse School of Medicine Board of Trustee minutes, Morehouse School of Medicine Archives, for a discussion of the ideal candidate for the presidency.

36. John E. Maupin Jr., interview with Marybeth Gasman, Apr. 10, 2009.

37. John E. Maupin Jr., interview with Marybeth Gasman, Apr. 10, 2009.

38. John E. Maupin Jr., interview with Marybeth Gasman, Apr. 10, 2009. See also Cohen, *Leadership and Ambiguity*, for a discussion of a president's leadership team.

39. John E. Maupin Jr., interview with Marybeth Gasman, Apr. 10, 2009.

40. John E. Maupin Jr., interview with Marybeth Gasman, Apr. 10, 2009.

41. John E. Maupin Jr., interview with Marybeth Gasman, Apr. 10, 2009; James Goodman, interview with Marybeth Gasman, Apr. 20, 2009.

42. John E. Maupin Jr., interview with Marybeth Gasman, Apr. 10, 2009; James Goodman, interview with Marybeth Gasman, Apr. 20, 2009.

43. John E. Maupin Jr., interview with Marybeth Gasman, Apr. 10, 2009.

44. Ibid.

45. Cohen, *Leadership and Ambiguity*; Weill, *Out in Front*.

46. Mary Kay Murphy, interview with Marybeth Gasman, Apr. 7, 2008. See also Morehouse School of Medicine fundraising materials, available from the Office of Institutional Advancement.

47. Mary Kay Murphy, interview with Marybeth Gasman, Apr. 7, 2008.

48. Mary Kay Murphy, interview with Marybeth Gasman, Apr. 7, 2008. See also Walton and Gasman, *Philanthropy, Volunteerism, and Fundraising*.

Chapter 8 · Nurturing Students

1. Walter Sullivan, interview with Marybeth Gasman, July 23, 2008.

2. Marjorie Smith, interview with Marybeth Gasman, Feb. 25, 2008; Fitzhugh Mullan, Candice Chen, Stephen Petterson, Gretchen Kolsky, and Michael Spagnola, "The Social Mission of Medical Education: Ranking the Schools," *Annals of Internal Medicine*, vol. 125, no. 12 (2010), 804–812.

3. Dan Blumenthal, interview with Marybeth Gasman, Feb. 10, 2008; Mullan et al., "Social Mission."

4. Dan Blumenthal, interview with Marybeth Gasman, Feb. 10, 2008.

5. Mullan et al., "Social Mission," 809.

6. Lonnie Boaz, interview with Marybeth Gasman, July 23, 2008.

7. Laura Perna, Valerie Lundy Wagner, Noah D. Drezner, Marybeth Gasman, Susan Yoon, Enakshi Bose, and Shannon Gary, "The Contributions of Historically Black Colleges and Universities to the Preparation of African American Women for STEM Careers: A Case Study," *Research in Higher Education*, vol. 50, no. 1 (2009), 1–23. See also Henry Drewry and Humphrey Doermann, *Stand and Prosper: Private Black Colleges and Universities* (Princeton, NJ: Princeton University Press, 1999); Marybeth Gasman and Christopher Tudico, *Historically Black Colleges and Universities: Triumphs, Troubles, and Taboos* (New York: Palgrave Macmillian, 2009).

8. Perna et al., "Contributions of Historically Black Colleges." See also Drewry and Doermann, *Stand and Prosper*.

9. Lonnie Boaz, interview with Marybeth Gasman, July 23, 2008.

10. Marjorie Smith, interview with Marybeth Gasman, Feb. 25, 2008.

11. Doug Paulsen, interview with Marybeth Gasman, June 14, 2008. Paulsen's attitude is quite common at Black colleges and universities, with myriad research studies demonstrating the commitment of faculty and the supportive atmosphere of the schools. See Gasman and Tudico, *Historically Black Colleges*; Drewry and Doermann, *Stand and Prosper*.

12. Doug Paulsen, interview with Marybeth Gasman, June 14, 2008.

13. Gasman and Tudico, *Historically Black Colleges*. See also Drewry and Doermann, *Stand and Prosper*.

14. Wayne Riley, interview with Marybeth Gasman, June 10, 2008.

15. Doug Paulsen, interview with Marybeth Gasman, June 14, 2008. See also Drewry and Doermann, *Stand and Prosper*.

16. Wayne Riley, interview with Marybeth Gasman, June 10, 2008; Mullan et al., "Social Mission." See also Drewry and Doermann, *Stand and Prosper*.

17. Angela Franklin, interview with Marybeth Gasman, June 14, 2008. See also Marjorie Smith, interview with Marybeth Gasman, Feb. 25, 2008.

18. Angela Franklin, interview with Marybeth Gasman, June 14, 2008.

19. Lonnie Boaz, interview with Marybeth Gasman, July 23, 2008.

20. Angela Franklin, interview with Marybeth Gasman, June 14, 2008.

21. Angela Franklin, interview with Marybeth Gasman, June 14, 2008; Lonnie Boaz, interview with Marybeth Gasman, July 23, 2008; Wayne Riley, interview with Marybeth Gasman, June 10, 2008.

22. Wayne Riley, interview with Marybeth Gasman, June 10, 2008.

23. Lonnie Boaz, interview with Marybeth Gasman, July 23, 2008.

24. Wayne Riley, interview with Marybeth Gasman, June 10, 2008.

25. Wayne Riley, interview with Marybeth Gasman, June 10, 2008.

26. Marjorie Smith, interview with Marybeth Gasman, Feb. 25, 2008. See also Lonnie Boaz, interview with Marybeth Gasman, July 23, 2008; Wayne Riley, interview with Marybeth Gasman, June 10, 2008; Angela Franklin, interview with Marybeth Gasman, June 14, 2008.

27. Lonnie Boaz, interview with Marybeth Gasman, July 23, 2008. In a study of

Spelman College, we found a similar atmosphere and attitude. See Perna at al., "Contributions of Historically Black Colleges."

28. Lonnie Boaz, interview with Marybeth Gasman, July 23, 2008.

29. Perna et al., "Contributions of Historically Black Colleges"; Mullan et al., "Social Mission."

30. Lonnie Boaz, interview with Marybeth Gasman, July 23, 2008; Wayne Riley, interview with Marybeth Gasman, June 10, 2008; Angela Franklin, interview with Marybeth Gasman, June 14, 2008.

31. Lonnie Boaz, interview with Marybeth Gasman, July 23, 2008.

32. Walter Sullivan, interview with Marybeth Gasman, July 23, 2008.

33. Walter Sullivan, interview with Marybeth Gasman, July 23, 2008.

Conclusion

1. Andrew Young, interview with Marybeth Gasman, June 8, 2008.

2. American Medical Association website, www.ama.org, accessed Nov. 11, 2009; Carrie Dumas, interview with Marybeth Gasman, Apr. 7, 2009.

3. Institute of Medicine, *Medical Education and Societal Needs: A Planning Report for the Health Professions* (Washington, DC: National Academy Press, July 1983); Sullivan Commission, *Missing Persons: Minorities in the Health Professions; A Report of the Sullivan Commission on Diversity in the Healthcare Workforce* (Washington, DC: U.S. Department of Health and Human Services, 2004).

4. Joe Frank Harris, interview with Marybeth Gasman, July 17, 2008.

5. See, for example, Jacqueline Fleming, *Blacks in College* (San Francisco: Jossey-Bass, 1984).

6. Fleming, *Blacks in College.*

7. Sullivan Commission, *Missing Persons*, 16–17.

8. Louis W. Sullivan, interview for Morehouse School of Medicine Public Relations Department, 2007, in the possession of the Public Relations Department, Morehouse School of Medicine, Atlanta, Georgia.

9. Louis W. Sullivan, interview with Marybeth Gasman, Feb. 13, 2009; David Satcher, interview with Marybeth Gasman, Apr. 8, 2008.

10. National Institutes of Health website, www.nih.gov, accessed Nov. 10, 2009.

11. Institute of Medicine website, www.iom.edu, accessed Nov. 11, 2009.

12. For a detailed description of this latter trend in Stanford University's medical school and its evolving mission—going from teaching to research—see Larry Cuban, *How Scholars Trumped Teachers: Change Without Reform in University Curriculum, Teaching, and Research, 1890–1990* (New York: Teachers College Press, 1999).

13. James H. Jones, *Bad Blood: The Tuskegee Syphilis Experiment* (New York: Free Press, 1981).

14. Louis W. Sullivan, interview for Morehouse School of Medicine Public Relations Department, 2007, Public Relations Department, Morehouse School of Medicine; Marlene Goldman, "The Grady Crunch," *Momentum* (Woodruff Health Sciences Center, Emory University), vol. 3, no. 1 (Winter 2000), 1–15.

15. Goldman, "Grady Crunch."

16. Craig Schneider, "Grady Memorial Hospital: Departing CEO May Get Big Payoff," *Atlanta Journal-Constitution*, July 9, 2008.

17. Ibid.; Goldman, "Grady Crunch."

18. Marybeth Gasman and Sibby Anderson-Thompkins, *Fund Raising from Black College Alumni: Successful Strategies for Supporting Alma Mater* (Washington, DC: Council for the Support and Advancement of Education [CASE], 2003); Andrea Walton and Marybeth Gasman, *Philanthropy, Volunteerism, and Fundraising in American Higher Education* (New York: Pearson, 2008).

19. Sullivan Commission, *Missing Persons*.

20. Council on Graduate Medical Education, *Minorities in Medical Education* (Washington, DC: Council on Graduate Medical Education, 1998), 4.

21. Ibid.

Appendix · Alumni Carrying Out the Mission

1. Mary Kay Murphy, interview with Marybeth Gasman, Apr. 7, 2009; Morehouse School of Medicine alumni marketing materials, 2008.

2. Bayou Clinic website, accessed Nov. 1, 2008; Louisiana Public Broadcasting website, accessed Nov. 1, 2008.

3. Marybeth Gasman, Benjamin Baez, Noah Drezner, Katherine Sedgwick, and Christopher Tudico, "Historically Black Colleges and Universities: Recent Trends," *Academe* (Jan.–Feb. 2007), 69–77.

4. Bayou Clinic website, accessed Nov. 1, 2008; Institute of Medicine of the National Academies of Science website, 2003, accessed Nov. 1, 2008; Speakers on Healthcare website, accessed Nov. 1, 2008.

5. Speakers on Healthcare website, accessed Nov. 1, 2008.

6. Bayou Clinic website, accessed Nov. 1, 2008; Speakers on Healthcare website, accessed Nov. 1, 2008.

7. Mary Kay Murphy, interview with Marybeth Gasman, Apr. 7, 2009; Morehouse School of Medicine Alumni marketing materials, 2008.

8. Speakers on Healthcare website, accessed Nov. 1, 2008.

9. Alabama Academy of Honor website, 2007, accessed Nov. 1, 2008.

10. Russ Willcutt, "Regina M. Benjamin: Bringing Health Care to People in Need," UAB [University of Alabama at Birmingham] Publications website, 2005, accessed Nov. 1, 2008; Mary Kay Murphy, interview with Marybeth Gasman, Apr. 7, 2009.

11. Bayou Clinic website, accessed Nov. 1, 2008.

12. Ibid.

13. Robert B. Baker, Harriet A. Washington, Ololade Olakanmi, Todd L. Savitt, Elizabeth A. Jacobs, Eddie Hoover, and Matthew K. Wynia, "African American Physicians and Organized Medicine, 1846–1968," *Journal of the American Medical Association*, vol. 300, no. 3 (2008), 306–313.

14. Willcutt, "Regina M. Benjamin."

15. Alabama Academy of Honor website, 2007, accessed Nov. 1, 2008; Bayou Clinic website, accessed Nov. 1, 2008.

16. Bayou Clinic website, accessed Nov. 1, 2008.

17. Alabama Academy of Honor website, 2007, accessed Nov. 1, 2008; American Hospital Association website, accessed Nov. 1, 2008; Nancy Shute, "America's Best Leaders: Regina Benjamin, Small-Town Primary Care Physician," *US News & World Report*, Nov. 19, 2008.

18. Alabama Academy of Honor website, 2007, accessed Nov. 1, 200.

19. Louisiana Public Broadcasting website, accessed Nov. 1, 2008.

20. American Hospital Association website, accessed Nov. 1, 2008.

21. Nicole Wallace, "MacArthur 2008 'Genius' Winners Include Urban Farmer and Rural Health Worker," *Chronicle of Philanthropy*, Sept. 23, 2008; Shute, "America's Best Leaders."

22. Louis W. Sullivan, interview with Marybeth Gasman, Feb. 13, 2009.

23. BNet Business Network website, 2007, accessed Nov. 1, 2008; MedeTel website, 2002, accessed Nov. 1, 2008; Thabiso Mochiko, "Agency Seeks Telephone Funds," 2005; Itumeleng Mogaki, "Telcos Should 'Go Extra Mile,'" *ITweb*, Mar. 10, 2005; Edward Webster, "Corporate Social Investment—Remote Counseling," *Business Day* (South Africa), Mar. 14, 2000, 22; Dejan Jovanovic, "SMEs Drive Telecoms for the Poor," *ITweb*, Nov. 24, 2004.

24. Lloyd Gedye, "USA-Microsoft partnership," *Mail & Guardian Online* (South Africa), Oct. 17, 2005.

25. B. Singh, "USA CEO steps down," *ITweb*, May 26, 2006.

26. *Citizen* (South Africa) website, accessed Nov. 1, 2008.

27. BNet Business Network website, 2007, accessed Nov. 1, 2008.

28. Ibid.

29. Meharry Medical College website, accessed Nov. 1, 2008; Wayne Riley, interview with Marybeth Gasman, June 14, 2008.

30. Meharry Medical College website, accessed Nov. 1, 2008.

31. Ibid.

32. Ibid.

33. Baylor College of Medicine website, accessed Nov. 1, 2008; Vanderbilt University School of Medicine website, accessed Nov. 1, 2008.

34. Vanderbilt University School of Medicine website, accessed Nov. 1, 2008.

35. Stephen J. Spann, "Report on Financing the New Model of Family Medicine," in "Task Force Report 6," a supplement to *Annals of Family Medicine*, vol. 2, no. 6 (Nov./Dec. 2004), S1–S21.

36. Ibid.

37. Joseph Conn and Jean DerGurahian, "Big Names, Numbers for HIMSS: Google Also Announces Major PHR Collaboration," *Modern Healthcare*, Mar. 3, 2008, 18; Jean DerGurahian, "States Take the Lead: While National Efforts to Standardize Patient-Safety Reporting Are Now Under Way, the States Remain Far Ahead of the Curve," *Modern Healthcare*, Dec. 10, 2007, 26; Society of Teachers of Family Medicine website, accessed

Nov. 1, 2008; Diana Manos, "Georgia Urges Physician Uptake of EHRs," *Healthcare IT News*, Mar. 31, 2008.

38. Healthcare Information and Management Systems Society website, accessed Nov. 1, 2008.

39. Alisa Ulferts, "Lives Hinge on Budget Choices," *St. Petersburg* (FL) *Times*, Jan. 20, 2003, 1B; Alisa Ulferts, "Health Cost Crises; Life Line for the Medically Needy," *St. Petersburg* (FL) *Times*, Apr. 22, 2003, 5B.

40. Mary Kay Murphy, interview with Marybeth Gasman, Apr. 7, 2009.

41. Morehouse School of Medicine website, 2007, accessed Nov. 1, 2008.

42. Abbott L. Ferriss, "Children in Poverty in Georgia," 2009, *New Georgia Encyclopedia* website.

43. Bainbridge, Georgia, website, accessed Nov. 1, 2008.

44. Kaufmann Clinic website, accessed Nov. 1, 2008.